起死回生

Qǐ Sǐ Huí Shēng

Raising the Dead and Returning Life:
Emergency Medicine of the
Qīng Dynasty

Excerpts from 《驗方新編》 *Yàn Fāng Xīn Biān*
(New Compilation of Proven Formulas),
by 鮑相璈 Bào Xiāng'áo

Lorraine Wilcox, L.Ac., Ph.D.

The Chinese Medicine Database
www.cm-db.com
Portland, Oregon

Raising the Dead and Returning Life:
Emergency Medicine of the Qīng Dynasty

起死回生

Qǐ Sǐ Huí Shēng

Lorraine Wilcox

Copyright © 2012 The Chinese Medicine Database

1017 SW Morrison #306
Portland, OR 97205 USA

COMP designation original Chinese work and English translation

Cover art courtesy of Michael Riley
Cover Design by Jonathan Schell L.Ac.
Library of Congress Cataloging-in-Publication Data:

Bao, Xiang'ao, fl.
    [Raising the Dead and Returning Life: Emergency Medicine of the Qīng Dynasty. English]
    Qi Si Hui Sheng = Raising the Dead and Returning Life.
    / translation Lorraine Wilcox
        p. cm.
    Includes Index.
    ISBN 978-0-9799552-3-5 (alk. paper)
    Medicine, Chinese   I. Wilcox, Lorraine. II. Title: Raising the
    Dead and Returning Life: Emergency Medicine of the Qīng Dynasty.

International Standard Book Number (ISBN): 978-0-9799552-3-5
Printed in the United States of America

Contents

Translation

9

Appendices

Indices

起
死
回
生

Introduction

Raising the Dead and Returning Life: Emergency Medicine of the Qīng Dynasty is essentially a first aid manual based on the practices of the common people of Southern China during the mid-nineteenth century. This book discusses first aid for cases that seem hopeless, such as hangings, drowning, poisoning, freezing, lightning strikes and so forth. Besides this, it includes treatment for trauma, including beatings, caning, burns and scalds, and bites. It also gives prescriptions for tobacco, alcohol, and opium addiction or overdose. Towards the end of the book, the treatment and prevention of epidemic diseases is described, as well as *gǔ* toxins and unusual diseases.

The Genesis of *Raising the Dead*

Raising the Dead consists of excerpts from Volumes 12, 13, 15, and 16 of *Yàn Fāng Xīn Biān* (New Compilation of Proven Formulas), written by Bào Xiāngáo during the 清 Qīng Dynasty.[1] My publisher Jonathan Schell and I came upon *Proven Formulas* by accident. Some time ago, scholar and practitioner of canonical medicine,[2] Arnaud Versluys returned from Chéngdū with a box of old medical books that were given to him when someone cleaned out his house. Among them were several books from a fourteen-volume series called 《 醫學易知 》 *Yī Xué Yì Zhī* (Easily Understood Medicine) that was published in Shànghǎi in 1919 and 1920. One of the volumes, 《 急救易 知 》 *Jí Jiù Yì Zhī* (Easily Understood Emergency Treatment), seemed interest-

---

1. The title of that book will now be referred to as *Proven Formulas*.
2. 經方 *jīng fāng*, literally classical formulas or canonical formulas, refers to the medicine of 张仲景 Zhāng Zhòngjǐng as described in 《 傷寒論 》 *Shāng Hán Lùn* and 《 金匱要略 》 *Jīn Guì Yào Lüè*.

ing. There has not been much published in English on Chinese-style emergency medicine. Of course, in the old days, there was no 911 to call, no ambulance to take someone to the emergency room. People generally knew a basic level of first aid. Families collected remedies. Small town doctors treated these patients with local herbs.

In researching *Easily Understood Emergency Treatment*, we eventually found that almost the entire book was taken from *Proven Formulas*. The author or authors of *Easily Understood Emergency Treatment* simply copied the items on emergency medicine that they wanted and discarded the rest. As we looked through the earlier book, we realized than in many ways it was more interesting. The author, Bào Xiāng'áo, sometimes described the symptoms of a disease, discussed the mechanisms of the suggested treatment, added personal experience, or gave a case history that he had collected. These were usually removed from *Easily Understood Emergency Treatment*.

Eventually we decided to directly excerpt and translate sections of *Proven Formulas*, but following the general structure of *Easily Understood Emergency Treatment*. Occasionally *Easily Understood Emergency Treatment* added a few remedies from other sources and we kept some of these. When this occurs, it is noted in the text or in a footnote.

An Overview of the Source and its Author

New Compilation of Proven Formulas was written by 鮑相璈 Bào Xiāng'áo (also known as 鮑雲韶 Bào Yúnsháo) and published in 1846 (*bǐng wǔ* year of Emperor Dào Guāng's reign, *Qīng* dynasty). *Proven Formulas* was originally a sixteen volume book, but 梅啟照 Méi Qǐzhào increased it to twenty-four volumes later during the *Qīng* dynasty.

The author, Bào, was a *Qīng* government official who spent a lot of time in Guǎngxī province, in the south of China. Bào was originally from Shànhuà (in present day Chángshā, Húnán province).

Bào became interested in time-tested formulas that were used by the people in general, as opposed to the more scholarly court medicine. He felt people in certain localities did not have adequate access to effective formulas, and disliked that some doctors or families held onto secret prescriptions. In his introduction to *Proven Formulas*, Bào wrote:

凡人不能無病，病必延醫服藥。然醫有時而難逢，藥
有時而昂貴。富者固無慮此，貧者時有束手之憂。余
幼時，見人有良方，秘而不傳世，心竊鄙之。因立願
廣求，不遺餘力，或見於古今之載籍，或得之戚友之
傳聞，皆手錄之。

Ordinary mortals are unable to escape disease; they must send for the doctor and take medicine when sick. However, sometimes it is difficult to find a doctor and sometimes the medicine is quite expensive. The rich certainly do not need to worry about this but the hands of the poor are tied and filled with grief now and again... In my childhood, I saw people with effective formulas they kept secret without passing them on, and I have despised this in my heart. Because of this I have desired to search widely [for effective formulas], not regretting the extra work. Sometimes I saw [a treatment] in an ancient or modern book, sometimes I obtained one from the talk of friends or relatives; I recorded them all with my own hand.

Over the course of twenty years, Bào searched for effective folk prescriptions and secret formulas wherever he went. He gathered these together and arranged them by category in his book.

Proven Formulas covers a wide variety of medical topics, including internal and external medicine, gynecology, pediatrics, emergency treatment, traumatology, dietary therapy, and so forth. The treatment methods are also quite varied, with oral administration of herbal medicine, topical application, ironing, acupuncture and moxibustion, ear acupuncture, bloodletting, massage and manipulation, cupping, *guāshā*, even artificial respiration, and some magical remedies.

Bào's book contains more than 6,000 prescriptions and treatment methods. Most herbal formulas have very few ingredients (often three or less) so they are simple and easy. Many of the substances would be found in the kitchen or around the house. Because most of the recipes came from the common people, they were time-tested and effective, but also convenient, inexpensive, and easy to obtain, at least in southern China during the *Qīng* Dynasty. Today, some of these substances have become rare, endangered, and expensive. Others are hard to identify as they may only be known in a particular region. Many of these treatments were not recorded in any earlier books. They have practical value and deserve more research.

The type of formulas that Bào collected is especially suited for emergency treatments. In an emergency, speed is essential. Since the substances are usually around the house, and the formulas have few ingredients, they can be made quickly.

More on the Contents of *Raising the Dead*

Since *Raising the Dead and Returning Life* discusses acute cases and comes from a folk tradition, many of the treatments are procedures for rescue (first aid techniques). Others are simple formulas made from ingredients that would be around the house. The quick and simple formulas provide timely treatment during emergencies using whatever is near-by. As *Proven Formulas* states in the discussion of death from falls and crushing injuries, "Select what is at hand and use it." There is no time to go to the pharmacy, purchase a formula, come home, and cook it.

There are also more complicated formulas that may be made in advance, in order to be prepared for a crisis. Other multi-ingredient formulas are given for the recovery phase or for less urgent issues. Acupuncture is not mentioned in these selections although in one case the inside of the ear apex is poked with a fish bone. Moxibustion is only prescribed a couple of times.

We are told in the first chapter that we should always attempt to rescue a person, even if we think the victim is already dead: "Even if there is not the least bit of life force left in the victim, you should still do all that is humanly possible and heed the command of heaven. You cannot see death without trying to rescue the victim." We are warned a few times that someone who appears dead, even for a few days, may sometimes be brought back to life.

Note that many times in this book the author cautioned the reader to be sure we get the genuine ingredient. He said that stores often sell fake products. Counterfeit products must have been a big problem at the time.

起
死
回
生

Warnings

There is a lot of information in this book which is clinically useful today. But many of the remedies are no longer relevant in today's clinic for the following reasons:

- In urgent cases the patient should be taken to the hospital emergency room right away. Procedures from Western medicine, such as CPR or rescue breathing should be the first priority, for both legal and medical reasons.
- In some cases, the remedy is from an endangered or threatened species, or has other ethical or legal concerns. Examples include 麝香 *shè xiāng* (musk), opium ash, or opium poppy husks.
- Some of the medicine is considered to have too much toxicity for internal use today. A few examples are 雄黃 *xióng huáng* (realgar), turpentine oil, 朱砂 *zhū shā* (cinnabar), or 馬兜鈴 *mǎ dōu líng*.
- Sometimes the medicine is not considered acceptable or clean to modern people (for example: child's urine or stool, cock's comb blood, fish gall bladder, tar from inside a chimney, or fingernails.)
- In some cases, the medicine suggested is unknown or unavailable in the West today. An example is 灰麵 *huī miàn* (flour mixed with the juice of herbs), or even mud from inside a well.

You must use your judgment; do not blindly follow any of these treatments. You must follow the current local standard of care. You must judge the seriousness of the condition and respond appropriately, perhaps using Western first aid or calling the paramedics as needed. It is the reader's responsibility to determine what is suitable in each case, and neither the publisher nor the author shall be held accountable for your use of these methods.

Really, this book is offered for historical understanding. You can extract a few treasures for the clinic, but when in doubt, follow the current standard of care, not what is in this book. Still, this volume can be mined to uncover many gems.

In most of our modern textbooks, Chinese emergency medicine is barely touched upon. Here is an opportunity to see how the ancient Chinese people managed emergency cases.

Terminology and Measurements

This is not a complete glossary, but these are a few terms that have specific meanings and need to be defined or differentiated from each other.

Taking medicine internally

服	*fú*	take orally/internally, a dose of internal medicine. In this translation when it says to take something or to give something, it means to take it orally.
灌	*guàn*	pour a liquid in (the nose or mouth) – when the patient is not fully conscious
沖服	*chōng fú*	drench a powder with a liquid and take it, dregs and all. This is sometimes called a draft or draught.
吹	*chuī*	to blow, often through a tube, into the orifices. Sometimes an herbal powder is blown in; occasionally it is just air.

External application

敷	*fū*	apply (an ointment, powder, etc.) externally. In this translation, when it says to apply something, it means to externally apply it to the affected site.
搽	*chá*	rub in (an ointment, powder, etc.)
貼	*tiē*	stick something (such as a plaster) on a site
塗	*tú*	smear something on a site
擦	*cā*	rub or wipe a site, perhaps with fresh ginger
掺	*chān*	sprinkle a powder on a site
滴	*dī*	to drip a liquid on a site or into the eyes

External heat therapy

| 熨 | *yùn* | iron (rub, press, or place an herbal hot pack on the body) |
| 熏 | *xūn* | fume, fumigate (make smoke reach an area) |

| 蒸 | zhēng | steam (make steam reach an area) |
| 灸 | jiǔ | moxibustion |

Miscellaneous

| 蟲 | chóng | bugs – includes worms, insects, spiders, snakes, reptiles, amphibians, larvae, etc., any creepy-crawly creature, including mythological ones |
| 酒 | jiǔ | translated here as liquor. It is often translated as wine, but that brings to mind the image of grape wine. Grape wine is mentioned only once in this volume. This term most often refers to distilled liquor from grains. White liquor is usually made from sorghum or maize; yellow liquor is usually made from rice or millet. |

Liquid Measurements: These are not precise and use common household objects. They are listed in order from largest to smallest, although the author may not have used these terms with precision.

碗	wǎn	bowl: a rice bowl, not a soup or noodle bowl
盃 or 杯	bēi	wine-cup: approximately the size of a small coffee mug
茶鍾	chá zhōng	tea cup: a Chinese tea cup
盞	zhǎn	small-cup: smaller and shallower than a tea cup
匙	chí	spoon: a Chinese soup spoon

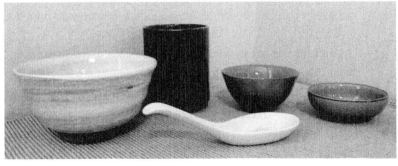

Liquid measurements

Back row, from left to right: bowl, wine-cup, tea cup, and small-cup.
In front: spoon.

起
死
回
生

Weights and Measures

Unit	Equivalent to	Metric Equivalent (during the *Qing* Dynasty)
1 斤 *jīn*	16 兩 *liǎng*	597 grams
1 兩 *liǎng*	10 錢 *qián*	37.3125 grams
1 錢 *qián*	10 分 *fēn*	3.7312 grams
1 分 *fēn*	10 釐 *lí*	0.3731 grams
1 釐 *lí*		0.0373 grams
1 合 *gě*		0.1035 liters
1 升 *shēng*	10 合 *gě*	1.0355 liters
1 斗 *dòu*	10 升 *shēng*	10.355 liters

A few other notes:

- When a recipe says to take a decoction cold, it means room temperature. Remember, they did not have refrigerators in 1846.
- Measurement of time: In ancient times, households did not have clocks. Cooking time was measured in different ways. These times are all approximate. The ancients were not obsessed with precision in timing the way modern people are. Examples of the way ancients described time:
  - 'Cook from ten cups down to seven' – instead of giving a length of time, cooking time is measured by the evaporation of liquid.
  - Rollings 滾 *gǔn*. For example, 'a hundred rollings.' This refers to the bubbling of a rolling boil. Probably a hundred rollings was a minute, give or take.
  - The time it takes to eat a meal, or the time it takes to walk three *lǐ*, or some other common activity.

Acknowledgements

- I am thankful to Arnaud Versluys for bringing back a box of old books from Chéngdū and giving them to the Chinese Medicine Database. Thanks also to the donor in Chéngdū who gave this box of books to Arnaud.
- I am grateful to Jonathan Schell for suggesting this project to me and for all

his work turning the manuscript into a book.

- I am indebted to Yue Lu for all her guidance with the difficult Chinese phrases and for researching so many of my questions. I really put her through a lot of trouble. I could never have finished without her.
- I appreciate Jerome Jiang, who also helped with a few difficult passages, and Ioannis Solos who provided some historical background.

All errors in translation are mine.

起
死
回
生

Chapter 1

各種死亡 *Gè Zhǒng Sǐ Wáng*
Various Kinds of Death[1]

Translator's Note: This chapter is abridged from Volume 12 of the 《驗方新編》 *Yàn Fāng Xīn Biān* (New Compilation of Proven Formulas).

凡自刎、縊死、溺死及一切自盡等症，人多畏懼不救，亦有以為已死。不能復活者，不知救治；得法亦可回生，下列各方，果能如法施治，必有奇效。即使萬無生理，亦當盡人事而聽天命；不可見死而不救也。

Whenever someone cuts his own throat, hangs himself, drowns, or any other type of suicide – people often are afraid so they do not attempt to rescue the victim. Sometimes there are victims who are taken as already dead. They cannot be revived if you do not know first aid. If you have learned the techniques, you can still return them to life. If you are able to carry out treatment according to the different formulas listed below, it will be extraordinarily effective. Even if there is not the least bit of life force left in the victim, you should still do all that is humanly possible and heed the command of heaven. You cannot see death without trying to rescue the person.

1. While the title says *death*, this chapter describes loss of consciousness and other conditions that are life-threatening. It especially discusses cases where a lesser doctor might think it is too late to rescue the patient.

五絕 *Wǔ Jué*
The Five Expirations[2]

凡五絕卒死，急取韭菜搗汁灌鼻中。或加皂角末、麝香同灌，更為快捷。

Whenever the five expirations give rise to sudden death, quickly crush *jiǔ cài* to extract the juice and pour it into the victim's nose. It is even quicker if you add *zào jiǎo* powder and *shè xiāng*. Pour all of the ingredients[3] in together.

縊死 *Yì Sǐ*
Hangings

回生丹灌之立活，真良丹也。

When you pour *Huí Shēng Dān* into a hanging victim, he will immediately come back to life. This is truly a great elixir.[4]

又方：不可割斷繩索，急以衣裹手，緊抵肛門；若是婦女，則連前陰抵住。緩緩抱住解下，安被放倒。一人以手緊提其髮，不可使頭垂下；一人微微撚整喉嚨；一人擦按心胸，又輕輕摩其肚腹；一人摩擦手足，緩緩彎動，若已硬直，但漸漸強彎屈之。又用腳裹衣緊抵肛門前陰，不使洩氣。以兩人用竹管吹其兩耳，不可住口。

---

2. There are various lists of the five expirations; one includes hanging, drowning, freezing to death, being crushed to death, and death during oppressive ghost dreams. All of these and more are discussed in detail below.

3. 灌 *guàn* means pouring a medicine in through the nose or mouth of an incapacitated patient. This technique was used as far back as the time of《素問‧繆刺論篇第六十三》*Sù Wèn•Miù Cì Lùn Piān Dì Liù Shí Sān* (Plain Questions 63, Treatise on Cross Needling) which prescribes pouring medicine into an unconscious patient.

4. 回生丹 *Huí Shēng Dān* (Return to Life Elixir) is the first formula in the chapter on Traumatic Injuries. The full name is 回生第一仙丹 *Huí Shēng Dì Yī Xiān Dān* (Most Effective Elixir of the Immortals for Returning Life). See appendix on p. 196.

Another formula: Do not cut the rope. Quickly bind your hand with clothing and tightly support the anus. Support the anterior yīn at the same time if this is a woman. Little by little untie the victim while holding on to him, then place a quilt on the ground and lower the victim onto it. One person should tightly pull up the hair with his hand; do not let the head droop down. Another person should slightly twist[5] the head to adjust the angle of the neck. Another person should rub and press the heart region and chest, while lightly and gently rubbing the abdomen. Another person should massage the hands and feet, bending and moving them little by little; if they are already hard and straight, the rescuer should still gradually try to bend them. Someone should wrap one of their feet with clothing and tightly support the anus and anterior yīn with it; do not let the qì leak out. Two people should blow into both ears through a bamboo tube; they cannot stop blowing.[6]

或用雞冠血滴鼻中，男左女右（ 男用雄雞，女用雌雞 ）；如此一飯之久，即有氣從口出，不可鬆手。少頃，以淡薑湯或清粥與食，令潤咽喉，漸漸能動，乃止 。

Cock's comb blood can be dripped into the nose using the left nostril on males and the right on females[7] (use a rooster for males, a hen for females). If you do all this, qì[8] will come out of the mouth within the time it takes to eat a meal. You cannot relax your hands.[9] In a short while, feed him thin ginger broth or clear light congee to moisten his throat. Don't stop until he is gradually able to move.

凡縊死從早至晚，雖已冷，可活；自夜至早，稍覺難救。總之身體稍頓，心下微溫者，雖一日以上，若依此救法，多吹多摸，無不活者。勿謂已冷，忽略不救 。

Whenever someone was hanging from morning until evening, he can be revived, even if he is already cold; but someone who was hanging from night

---

5. Manipulate the head in order to straighten the spine.

6. *Sù Wèn*, Chapter 63 prescribes blowing into an unconscious patient's ears with bamboo tubes.

7. Left is yáng and is associated with males; right is yīn and corresponds to female.

8. Breath.

9. Don't stop working on the patient.

until morning is seen as a somewhat more difficult to rescue. In general, even if a day or more has passed, no one will not come back to life if you follow this rescue method, and use a lot of blowing and a lot of stroking – as long as the body is a little soft and is slightly warm below the heart. Do not say: "he is already cold," and fail to rescue him because of neglect.

或再將其兩手大拇指，並排平正，以小帶縛定，於兩指縫中離指甲角一分半之處，名鬼哭穴，用艾火燒三七次；並燒兩腳心三次，即活。凡無故中邪而自縊者，以多燒鬼哭穴為要。

Both of the patient's thumbs can also be placed side by side, level with each other and bound together securely with a small ribbon. The site called Ghost Crying Points (*Guǐ Kū Xué*) is on the 'seam' between the two thumbs, 1.5 *fēn* from the corner of the nail. Burn mugwort fire: three times seven cones, and at the same time, burn moxibustion on the hearts of the two feet: three cones. The patient will then come back to life. It is important to burn a lot of moxibustion on the Ghost Crying Points whenever evil strikes and someone hangs himself without reason.

又方：炒熱生鹽二大包，從頸喉熨至臍下，冷則隨換，不可住手，其痰盡下；並用人對口以氣灌之，其活更快。

Another formula: Stir-fry two large bundles of unprocessed salt until hot. Iron[10] the patient from the neck and throat to below the umbilicus. When the salt is cold, exchange it [for the other bundle of hot salt]. You cannot stop moving your hands. His phlegm will completely move downward. At the same time, have someone pour qì [air, breath] into his mouth, which will make his revival even more rapid.

又方：陳皮（八分）、厚朴、製半夏（各一錢）、肉桂、乾薑（各五分）、甘草（三分），右水煎服。

Another formula:

chén pí	陳皮	8 *fēn*

---

10. 熨 *yùn* (ironing) is an ancient technique in which a hot substance is rubbed or pressed into the body.

hòu pò	厚朴	1 *qián*
zhì bàn xià	製半夏	1 *qián*
ròu guì	肉桂	5 *fēn*
gān jiāng	乾薑	5 *fēn*
gān cǎo	甘草	3 *fēn*

Boil the above in water and give it to the patient internally.

溺水死 Nì Shuǐ Sǐ
Drowning

撈起時，急將口撬開，橫唧筯一根，使可出水。以竹管吹其兩耳。碾生半夏末如豆大，吹其鼻孔；又用皂角末置管中，吹其穀道。

When the victim is dredged up out of the water, quickly force his mouth open to let the water out and place a chopstick in it horizontally. Blow into both ears through a bamboo tube. Grind *shēng bàn xià* into a powder and blow a pile the size of a bean into his nostrils. *Zào jiǎo* powder can also be put into a tube and blown into his grain path [anus].

如係夏月，將溺人肚腹，橫覆牛背之上，兩邊使人扶住，牽牛緩緩而行，腹中之水，自然從口中並大小便流出。再用生薑湯調蘇合丸灌之；或生薑汁灌之，並用生薑擦牙。

If the drowning occurred during the summer months, drape the victim across the back of an ox, belly-down. Have people support him on both sides, while leading the ox so that it walks slowly. The water in the abdomen will naturally flow out from his mouth and with his stool and urine. Then mix *Sū Hé Wán*[11] with decocted *shēng jiāng* and pour it into the patient. Some pour in *shēng jiāng* juice and rub his teeth with *shēng jiāng* at the same time.

若無牛，用一人覆臥躬腰，令溺人如前，將肚腹橫覆於活人身上，令活人微微搖動，水亦可出；或用大鍋一口，覆寬櫈上，將溺人覆於鍋上，亦可。

---

11. See appendix on p. 196.

27

If an ox is not available, have someone bend at the waist and drape the victim over him as before [in the method with the ox]. Let the victim's belly lie across the body of the living person, and have the living person gently rock back and forth. The water will still come out. An upside-down cauldron can also be placed on a broad bench and the drowning victim can be draped over the cauldron.

如係冬月，即將溼衣更換；一面炒鹽，用布包熨臍；一面厚鋪被褥，取竈內草灰，多鋪被褥之上，令溺人覆臥於上，臍下墊棉枕；一面，仍以草灰將全身厚蓋之，灰上再加被褥，不可使灰瞇於眼內。按灰性暖而能拔水。凡蒼蠅溺水死者，以灰埋之，少頃即活，此明驗也。

If the drowning occurred during the winter months, change the victim's wet clothing. Wrap stir-fried salt in cloth and iron his umbilicus with it. Then lay out thick bedding and spread a lot of plant ash from inside the stove on it. Lay the drowning victim face down on top [of the ash], and place a cotton pillow beneath his umbilicus. Then cover his entire body with a thick layer of plant ash as before, and pile more bedding on top of the ash. Do not let the ash get into the eyes. Note that the nature of ash is warm and it is able to pull out water. Whenever you cover a drowned housefly with ash, it will come back to life in a little while. This explains the experience.

其撬口啣箸、灌蘇合丸、生薑湯，吹耳、鼻、穀道等事，俱照夏日法。冬日醒後，宜少飲湯酒；夏日宜少飲粥湯。

The activities such as prying open the mouth and holding a chopstick in it; pouring in *Sū Hé Wán* and *shēng jiāng* decoction; blowing into the ears, nose, and grain path [anus] are all summertime method. In the wintertime, the victim should drink a little soup and liquor after reviving. In summertime, the victim should drink a little congee and soup.

溺人倘或微笑，必急掩其口鼻，如不掩住，則笑不可止，不能救矣；又不可急於見火，一見必大笑而死。

If the drowning victim smiles, quickly shield his mouth and nose. If it is not covered, his laughter cannot stop and you will be unable to save him. You also cannot be quick to expose him to fire. As soon as he catches sight of fire, he will laugh loudly and then die.

又以酒罈一個，紙片一把，燒放罈內，急以罈口覆臍上，冷即燒紙片放罈內，覆臍，去水即活。

A burning strip of paper can also be placed inside a liquor jug, then quickly cover his umbilicus with the opening. When it is cold, quickly place another burning strip of paper inside the jar and cover his umbilicus again. When the water is removed, he will live.

又初救起時，尚有微氣，或胸前尚煖，速令生人脫貼身熱衣，為之更換。

Also at the time of the initial rescue, if there is still a small amount of qì – perhaps the front of the chest is still warm – quickly have a living person take off the warm clothing from next to his skin and exchange it with the patient's [wet clothing].

抱擔身上，將屍微微倒側之，令其腹內水流出，若水往外，即有生機；一面用粗紙燒煙熏鼻，稍熏片時，即用皂角研細末，吹入鼻竅，但得微有噴嚏，即可得生。

Hold the victim's body over someone's shoulder, and slightly turn the 'corpse' upside down and side to side. Make the water in his abdomen come out. If the water comes out, there is a better chance at survival. Simultaneously burn coarse paper and fumigate his nose with the smoke. Lightly fumigate him for a moment, and then blow finely-powdered *zào jiǎo* into his nostrils. The victim will live if he sneezes slightly.

又灌酒湯，不可太熱，恐傷齒盡落。

Also pour boiled liquor into him. It cannot be too hot or else it will damage his teeth and they will all fall out.

凍死 *Dòng Sǐ*
Freezing to Death

冬月凍極之人，雖人事不知，但胸前有微溫，皆可救 。倘或微笑，必為急掩其口鼻，否則不救；又不可驟令近火，見火必大笑而死 。

The winter months may freeze people to the extreme. Even if unconscious, they can all be saved as long as the front of the chest is slightly warm. If the patient smiles, quickly shield his mouth and nose; otherwise, he cannot be saved. Neither can the patient be abruptly taken near a fire. If he sees fire, he will laugh loudly and then die.

凍死，四肢直，口噤，有微氣者，用生半夏末如豆大少許，入耳鼻內；又用大鍋炒灰，布包，熨心腹上，冷則換之；候目開，以溫酒及清粥少少與之，不可太熱，恐傷齒盡落；如已救活，用生薑（ 搗碎 ）、陳皮（ 搥碎 ）各等分，用水三碗，煎一碗，溫服 。

In freezing to death, the four limbs are straight and the mouth is clenched. If there is slight qì [breath, warmth], put a pile of *shēng bàn xià* powder about the size of a bean inside his ears and nose. Also stir-fry ashes in a cauldron, wrap them in cloth, and iron his heart region and abdomen. When it becomes cold, exchange it [for a hot one]. Wait for his eyes to open, then give him warm liquor and thin clear congee little by little. It cannot be too hot or else you will damage his teeth and they will all fall out. Once he is revived, boil equal portions of *shēng jiāng* (crushed) and *chén pí* (beaten into pieces) in three bowls of water until one bowl is left. The patient should take it warm.

壓死跌死 *Yā Sǐ Diē Sǐ*
Crushed to Death or Falling to One's Death

急扶起，盤腳坐地，以手提其髮 。將生半夏末（ 約豆大 ）吹兩鼻中，以生薑汁灌之 。苟心頭微溫，雖一日亦活 。再用白糖調水與服，散其瘀血；或加童便灌之 。

Quickly help the victim up. Bend his legs so he is sitting on the ground [cross-legged]. Raise his hair with your hands [to hold his head up]. Blow *shēng bàn xià* powder (a pile about the size of a bean) into both of his nostrils. Pour *shēng jiāng* juice into him. Even if a day has already passed, if his heart region and head are slightly warm, he can still return to life. Then give him a dose of white sugar mixed with water. This will scatter the blood stasis. Some add *tóng biàn* (child's urine) and pour it into him.

又方：回生丹灌之立活。

Another formula: Pour *Huí Shēng Dān* into him.[12] He will immediately come to life.

雷擊死 *Léi Jī Sĭ*
Death by Lightning Strike

蚯蚓搗融，敷臍上，半日即活；或回生丹灌之，亦妙。

Pound *qiū yīn* (earthworms) until soft and apply them to the umbilicus. He will come back to life in half a day. It is also wonderful to pour *Huí Shēng Dān* into him.

睡魘死 *Shuì Yǎn Sĭ*
Death from Oppressive Ghost Dreams during Sleep

原有燈，即存燈；無燈，切不可用燈照。急用生半夏末（約一豆大）吹入兩鼻；取母雞冠血搽面上，乾則再搽，即醒。

If the light was already on, leave it on. If there was no light, be sure not to turn it on. Quickly blow *shēng bàn xià* powder (a pile about the size of a bean) into both nostrils, and then rub blood from a hen's comb onto his face. When it dries, rub it in again, and then he will wake up.

---

12. *Huí Shēng Dān* (Return to Life Elixir) is described in the chapter on Traumatic Injuries below on p. 111.

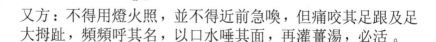

又方：不得用燈火照，並不得近前急喚，但痛咬其足跟及足大拇趾，頻頻呼其名，以口水唾其面，再灌薑湯，必活。

Another formula: You must not use a lamp for illumination nor call out urgently near the patient. However, bite the victim's heels and big toes to cause him pain and call his name repeatedly. Spit saliva on his face[13] and then pour ginger decoction into him. He will come back to life.

又方：酒調蘇合丸，灌之。

Another formula: Pour liquor mixed with *Sū Hé Wán* into the patient.

又方：用艾燒兩足大拇指向上生毛處三七次；或燒鬼哭穴亦可。

Another formula: Burn three times seven mugwort cones on the top of both big toes where the hairs grow. You can also burn it on the Ghost Crying Points.

治夢魘 *Zhì Mèng Yǎn*
Treating Oppressive Ghost Dreams

大塊明雄（硃砂更妙）戴頭上，並繫左腋下，可免鬼魅，並解惡夢。

Put a big lump of *míng xióng* (*zhū shā* is even more wonderful) on the victim's head and at the same time bind one to his left armpit. This can ward off ghosts and goblins, resolving nightmares[14] at the same time.

中邪死 *Zhòng Xié Sǐ*
Death from Evil Strike

生半夏末如豆大，各吹兩鼻中；燒炭一爐，以陳醋潑炭上，使患者聞得醋氣，即活。須捉其兩手，勿令驚。或灌醋於鼻

---

13. In Chinese folk tales, ghosts are afraid of spit.
14. Literally 'malign dreams.'

內，或用樟木燒煙熏之亦可。

Blow a pile of *shēng bàn xià* powder the size of a bean into both nostrils. Sprinkle mature vinegar on burning charcoal in a stove, and make the patient smell the vinegar qì [odor], which will bring him back to life. Then grasp both his hands. Do not startle him. Some pour vinegar into his nose. *Zhāng mù* can also be burned to fumigate him with the smoke.

鬼打死 *Guǐ Dǎ Sǐ*
Beat to Death by a Ghost

睡魔死、中邪死、俱可用此方。白毛烏骨雞血搽胸前，並將雞煮湯灌之，極效。

This formula can be used for death from oppressive ghost dreams or death from evil strike. Rub blood from a chicken with white feathers and black bones and skin into the front of the chest. At the same time, make broth from the chicken and pour it into him. This is extremely effective.

驚嚇死 *Jīng Xià Sǐ*
Frightened to Death

回生丹灌之，立活。

Pour *Huí Shēng Dān* into the patient,[15] which will immediately bring him back to life.

又方：醇酒一二杯，溫熱灌之，自活；或用生半夏末（一豆大）吹兩鼻中，亦可。

Another formula: Pour one or two cups of warm good quality liquor (*chún jiǔ*) into the patient, which will automatically bring him back to life. You can also blow *shēng bàn xià* powder, (a pile the size of a bean) into both nostrils.

---

15. *Huí Shēng Dān* is the first formula in the chapter on Traumatic Injuries on p. 111.

痰厥死 *Tán Jué Sǐ*
Death due to Phlegm Reversal

巴豆搗爛，綿紙包，板壓取油，作撚燒煙，熏鼻中，片刻，
吐出痰血，即愈；或用生半夏末如豆大，吹兩鼻中。

Pound *bā dòu* to a pulp. Wrap it in tissue paper and press it with a board to remove the oil. Twist the paper around it, roast it until smoking, and fume the patient's nose. In a short while he will vomit out blood and phlegm, and then he will recover. Some blow a pile of powdered *shēng bàn xià* the size of a bean into both nostrils.

氣厥死 *Qì Jué Sǐ*
Death due to Qì Reversal

照上痰厥方治之。

Treat it according to the above formula for phlegm reversal.

中風死 *Zhòng Fēng Sǐ*
Death by Wind Stroke

亦可照上痰厥方治之。

This can also be treated according to the above formula for phlegm reversal.

尸厥死 *Shī Jué Sǐ*
Death due to Corpse Reversal

由入廟、吊喪得者。附子（七錢重者，泡熱，去皮臍，為
末），右分二服，每服酒三盞，煎一盞；如無附子，生薑汁
半盞，和酒同煎百滾，連灌二服，即醒；或照上痰厥方，亦
可。

This comes from entering a temple or making a condolence call. *Fù zǐ* (seven *qián* in weight, soak it in hot [water],[16] remove the skin and the 'umbilicus,' and powder it). Divide the above into two doses. The patient should take each dose boiled in three small-cups of liquor down to one small-cup. If you do not have *fù zǐ*, use a half of a small-cup of ginger juice. Blend it with liquor and boil them together for a hundred 'rollings.'[17] When you pour in two consecutive doses, he will wake up. This can also be treated according to the above formula for phlegm reversal.

尸厥死腹響如雷 *Shī Jué Sǐ Fù Xiǎng Rú Léi*
Death due to Corpse Reversal with Thunderous Abdominal Sounds

硫黄（一兩）、焰硝（五錢），右研細，分作三服，好酒煎至煙起為止，候溫，灌下片時，再服，即安。

Finely grind *liú huáng* (one *liǎng*) and *yàn xiāo* (five *qián*). Divide it into three doses. Boil it in good liquor, stopping when steam[18] arises. Wait for it to be warm [not hot] and pour it down in a moment. He will be secure when you give him another dose or two.

忽然胡言亂語昏迷跌倒
Hū Rán Hú Yán Luàn Yǔ Hūn Mí Diē Dǎo
Sudden Raving and Falling Down in a Stupor

此症不省人事，切勿挪動；動則難治。急用大爆竹放頭腳兩處（頭頂邊一個，腳底一個），一齊點放，其人自醒，大小皆治，屢試如神。

---

16. This passage appears in a number of other books. In some cases the character 熱 *rè* (hot) is not there. In that case, it would read "soak it, remove the skin and 'umbilicus'…"

17. In ancient times, households did not have clocks so time was measured in other ways (the time it takes to eat a meal, or walk three *lǐ*, or boil down to 70%, or here, a hundred 'rollings.' This refers to the bubbling of a rolling boil.

18. It literally says 'smoke' here.

35

In this pattern there is loss of consciousness.[19] Be sure not to move the patient; it becomes difficult to treat when you move him. Quickly set off big firecrackers near both his head and feet (one at the side of the crown of his head and one at the soles of his feet). Set them off simultaneously, and the patient will automatically wake up. This treats both adults and children. It has been repeatedly tested and it works like a miracle!

暴厥死 *Bào Jué Sǐ*
Death due to Sudden Reversal

凡人卒然倒仆，急扶入煖室，扶住正坐；用火炭沃醋，使醋氣沖入鼻中，良久自醒；或搗韭菜汁灌鼻；或用皂角末吹鼻，得噴嚏，即醒。如倉卒無藥，急於人中穴及兩足大拇指離甲一韭葉許，各用艾火灸三五次，即活。

Whenever someone suddenly falls down, quickly help him into a warm house. Support him so he can sit upright. Moisten burning charcoal with vinegar, and make the vinegar qì [odor] rush into his nose. After a long time, he will automatically wake up. Some pound *jiǔ cài* into juice and pour it into his nose, while others blow *zào jiǎo* powder into his nose. He will wake up when he sneezes. If you are in a hurry and do not have these herbs, quickly apply moxibustion to Rén Zhōng (Du 26) and to the big toes, about a leek's distance from the nail; apply three times five cones of mugwort fire moxibustion on each site, and he will come back to life.

發花風死 *Fā Huā Fēng Sǐ*
Death from Flower Wind[20]

此症多死於牀上，急用麝香填入臍眼，加薑一片，蓋麝上，艾火灸，則生。

---

19. Literally 'unaware of human affairs.'

20. 花風 *huā fēng* (flower wind): This refers to someone collapsing in bed during sex. The image is of flower petals dispersing in the wind. Flowers contain the image of a beautiful woman. Dispersing in the wind holds the image of dissipation. Of course, wind diseases tend to have sudden onset.

This pattern often results in death in bed. Quickly insert *shè xiāng* into the 'eye' of the umbilicus. Cover the musk with a slice of ginger, and the patient will live when you apply mugwort fire moxibustion on top.

起
死
回
生
·
一

Chapter 2

服毒 *Fú Dú*
Poisoning

Translator's Note: This chapter is abridged from Volume 12 of 《驗方新編》 *Yàn Fāng Xīn Biān*. There, this chapter is part of the previous one and does not have a separate heading. General items that can cause toxicity or poisoning will be called by their common name. The Pīnyīn transliteration will be used for substances used in Chinese medicine. These substances are listed in the Appendix.

凡解毒藥，俱宜冷服；大忌飲熱湯水，飲熱則不可救；若見酒必死。

Whenever you use the various medicines to resolve toxins or poisoning,[21] they should be taken cold.[22] The great taboo is drinking hot decoctions, soup, or water. When a poisoning victim drinks hot liquids, he cannot be saved. If he is exposed to liquor, he will die.

解救百毒 *Jiě Jiù Bǎi Dú*
Resolving the Hundred Toxins

乾淨地上（黃土地更好）挖三尺深，入水一桶，用棍攪動，名曰地漿，能解百毒。

---

21. 毒 *dú* may be translated as toxin, toxins, toxic, poison, poisoning, venom, etc. depending on the context. It is all the same word in Chinese.

22. In books of this time period, taking a decoction cold actually means room temperature: letting the decoction cool off before taking it. It does not mean refrigerating the decoction.

Dig three *chǐ* deep into clean earth (*huáng tǔ dì* (yellow earth [loess] is the best). Add a bucket of water and stir it with a stick. This is called *Dì Jiāng* (Earth Slurry).[23] It can resolve the hundred toxins.

凡食隔夜菓餅菜蔬茶水酒漿等物，或飲田塘溪澗井溝之水，誤中無名百毒者，取飲數碗，極為神效。愈後戒食鱔魚。

Whenever someone is accidentally struck by the hundred nameless toxins – after eating things from the previous night, such as fruits and cakes, vegetables, tea water, or liquor; or after drinking water from a field dike, mountain stream, well, or ditch – drink several bowls [of *Dì Jiāng*]. It has extremely miraculous effects. After recovery, eating eel or fish is forbidden.

中毒七孔流血 *Zhòng Dú Qī Kǒng Liú Xuè*
Bleeding from the Seven Orifices due to Poisoning

刺蝟皮（煆存性），右為末，每服三錢，酒調下，立止。

Powder *cì wèi pí* (calcine preserving its nature).[24] Swallow three *qián* each dose mixed with liquor, and it will immediately stop.

解鴉片煙毒 *Jiě Yā Piàn Yān Dú*
Resolving Poisoning from Smoking Opium

急用活鴨血多多灌之，凡服鴉片煙者，最為神效。

Quickly pour a great deal of live duck blood into the victim. This is miraculously effective for anyone who takes opium.

---

23. 地漿 *Dì Jiāng* (Earth Slurry): A slurry is thin sloppy mud, or any fluid mixture of a pulverized solid with a liquid. Slurry is one of the meanings of 漿 *jiāng*. *Dì Jiāng* is very similar to a recipe in《五十二病方》*Wǔ Shí Èr Bìng Fāng* (Formulas for Fifty-Two Diseases), one of the 馬王堆 *Mǎwángduī* medical manuscripts of the early *Hàn* dynasty. In that book, it is indicated for 烏喙 *wū huì* (monkshead) poisoning.

24. 'Preserving its nature' means that the original properties are still present, so it is not calcined until the transformation is complete.

若身冷氣絕，似乎已死，如身體柔頓，則臟腑經絡之氣，尚在流通，實未死也，乃鴉片烈性醉迷之故耳。將其人放在潮溼陰地，用箸撬開牙齒（或用烏梅擦之亦開）以箸橫放口內，使口常開，以冷水時時灌之，或白沙糖調冷水灌之，更妙。

When the body is cold, qì has expired and the victim appears to be dead. If the body is still soft, the qì of the organs, channels, and network vessels is still circulating; the victim is not really dead yet. This is the result of being lost in strong opium intoxication. Place the person in a moist shaded cool place, and force his teeth open with chopsticks (some rub [his jaw] with *wū méi* and it will open). Place a chopstick horizontally inside his mouth to make it stay open, then constantly pour cold water into him. It is even more wonderful to mix white granulated sugar with cold water and pour it in.

外用手帕二三條，以冷水泡透，放胸前輪流更換，或用整塊豆腐亦可；又用冷水一盆，將頭髮散放盆內，時時換水；切不可見太陽，一見日照，即不可救。

Externally use two or three handkerchiefs that have been thoroughly soaked in cold water. Place one on the front of his chest and keep changing it; an entire block of tofu can be used instead. Also place his head hair into a basin of cold water, and change the water constantly. Be sure he is not exposed to the sun; as soon as he sees sunlight, he cannot be rescued.

三四日後，鴉片之氣，散盡即活，如身不硬，雖七日內亦可回生，切不可以為無救，遽行棺殮；此法無論服毒輕重，雖手足青黑，亦效。

After three or four days, when all the opium qì is dispersed, he will live. If his body is not hard he can still return to life, even if it has been up to seven days. Be sure not to take this type of case as impossible to rescue, by putting him in a coffin and grave clothes too quickly. This method is still effective, no matter what dose of poison, light or heavy, even if the hands and feet are bluish-black.

切忌灌服醬油，恐受鹽滷之毒，反致誤事；若服藥雜亂，亦不可救。活後多服白沙糖水，及生綠豆末，沖水服，最效。

By all means avoid pouring in or giving the patient soy sauce or else he will suffer from *Yán Lǔ* (bittern)[25] toxicity, resulting in a bungled treatment. If you give him herbs randomly, he cannot be saved. After he returns to life, he should take a lot of white granulated sugar in water. Taking fresh *lù dòu* powder drenched with water is quite effective.

又方：廣州產木棉花六錢撕鬆，用潔淨大瓦鉢將鐵火鉗叉開，架於鉢口，置棉鉗上，火燒淨煙，成灰，放在鉢內，加食鹽二錢，用木棍擂灰並鹽，成極細末，開水半碗，沖入鉢內，用手將鉢內四面之灰，洗入湯內，復用箸在鉢內調勻；連灰帶湯，概行服下，片刻煙毒即可吐出。

Another formula: Loosely rip apart six *qián* of *mù mián huā* that was produced in Guǎngzhōu.[26] Use a clean large tile earthenware basin. Open iron fire tongs and put them inside a basin. Hold the cotton with the tongs and set it on fire until it finishes smoking and becomes ash, then place the ash inside the basin. Add two *qián* of table salt, and pestle the ash and salt together with a wooden stick to make an extremely fine powder. Drench it with half a bowl of boiled water inside the basin. Use your hands to wash the ashes with the hot water, all around the inside the basin. Mix the ash and water inside the basin evenly again with chopsticks. Have the patient swallow it all down including the ash that is carried by the hot water. In a short while, the opium toxins will be vomited out.

吞煙至六七錢者，連灌此藥二副，三四刻許煙毒亦可嘔出；若吞至一兩零者，連灌此藥三副，藥性行到自能漸漸還陽，大吐而愈；閒有不吐者，則從大便瀉出，煙毒亦自解去。

If someone has swallowed up to six or seven *qián* of opium,[27] continuously pour two doses of this medicine into him. If you reach him within about three

---

25. 鹽滷 *yán lǔ* (bittern) is magnesium chloride. It is a white powder left over from seawater after the water has been evaporated and the sodium chloride (table salt) has been removed. It is sometimes used to curdle soy milk in order to make tofu. Perhaps this means a more general salt toxicity which can occur when water intake is limited and excessive salt is consumed. Since the patient has been unconscious for a while, he is probably dehydrated.

26. This refers to the naturally occurring cotton ball that grows after flowering is complete. It is then fluffed up to get more air inside so it will burn well.

27. This implies swallowing opium to attempt suicide.

or four quarter hours,[28] the opium toxins still can be vomited out. If the patient has swallowed up to one *liǎng* or a little more, continuously pour three doses of this medicine into him. When the effect of this medicine arrives, it is automatically able to return *yáng* little by little. He will recover after a lot of vomiting. If he does not vomit, it sometimes drains out through the stool [diarrhea]; the opium toxins will still automatically resolve and will be removed.

凡遇救人之際，不可慌亂，須照此方細心製之，果能製藥如法，無不神效 。

Whenever you rescue someone, you cannot be frantic. You must attentively prepare the medicine according to this formula. If you are able to prepare the medicine according to the instructions, it is invariably miraculous.

他如水粉鉛粉砒霜野菰諸毒，以此解救，亦皆神效；但僅用木棉燒灰，擂末，調開水服，不可用鹽 。

Use this [method] to rescue people from all the other poisons such as *shuǐ fěn*, *qiān fěn*,[29] *pī shuāng*, and *yě gū*; it is miraculously effective for them all. But only give them the *mù mián huā* reduced to ashes, pestled into a powder, and mixed with boiled water. You cannot use the salt [for these poisons].

又方：真南硼砂（ 黃色如膠者為真 ），右冷水調服，可以立解，試之屢有奇驗 。

Another formula: Mix genuine *nán péng shā* (the genuine kind is yellow-colored and glue-like)[30] with cold water and give it orally. This can also immediately resolve the toxins, and has been tested repeatedly with extraordinary efficacy.

---

28. It is not clear if this refers to quarters of a Western single-hour (fifteen minutes each) or quarters of a Chinese double-hour (thirty minutes each).

29. According to various sources, 水粉 *shuǐ fěn* is a synonym for 鉛粉 *qiān fěn*. However, *qiān fěn* is listed next. So it is unclear what the author meant. Perhaps he was just giving both names for the same substance.

30. 南硼砂 *nán péng shā* and 硼砂 *péng shā* both refer to borax. However, *nán péng shā* may be more yellow in color. Note that many times in this book the author cautions us to be sure we get the genuine ingredient. At times he tells us how stores sell a fake product. Counterfeit products must have been a big problem at the time.

又方：用清油灌之，立解，緣鴉片煙粘滯腸胃，見油即散也。

Another formula: It will immediately resolve when you pour clear oil[31] into the patient because opium smoke is sticky and stagnates in the intestines and stomach; it dissipates when it is exposed to oil.

解砒霜毒 Jiě Pī Shuāng Dú
Resolving White Arsenic Poisoning

防風（一兩）研末，冷水調服，或用四兩，冷水擂汁灌服，亦可，屢試如神。

Grind *fáng fēng* (one *liǎng*) into a powder. Mix it with cold water and give it orally. You can also pestle four *liǎng* of *fáng fēng* in cold water and pour the liquid in. This has been tried repeatedly and works like a miracle!

解野菌毒 Jiě Yě Jùn Dú
Resolving Wild Mushroom Poisoning

照前取地漿水三四碗，入喉即活，至神至妙，切勿輕視。亦不必用別藥（以鹽擦牛舌上，以碗盛牛涎灌之奇效）。

The patient should take three or four bowls of *Dì Jiāng* (Earth Slurry) water according to the directions above.[32] If it goes down the throat, he will live; this is extremely miraculous, extremely wonderful. Be sure not to take mushroom poisoning lightly. In addition, you must not use other herbs. (Rub salt onto the tongue of an ox and use a bowl to catch the ox saliva. Pouring this into the patient is extremely effective.)

起死回生 • 二

---

31. According to Wiseman, 清油 *qīng yóu* refers to soy sauce. According to other dictionaries, it may mean vegetable oil, tea oil or simply clear oil without sediments.

32. On p. 39.

解黄藤草毒 *Jiě Huáng Téng Cǎo Dú*
Resolving *Huáng Téng Cǎo* Poisoning

（ 即水莽草，或云即斷腸草 ）黑豆（ 一升 ）煮濃汁，候冷透，飲之，立解；或照前解斷腸草毒，均極效 。

(Meaning *shuǐ mǎng cǎo*, sometimes called *duàn cháng cǎo*.)[33] Boil black soybeans (one *shēng*) into a concentrated liquid. Wait until the liquid is thoroughly cold and have the patient drink it. It will immediately resolve the toxins. Some treat this according to the above formulas to resolve *duàn cháng cǎo* poisoning, which is just as effective.

解野草毒 *Jiě Yě Cǎo Dú*
Resolving Weed[34] Poisoning

照上解斷腸草各方治之；或飲甘草水，或飲地漿，均效 。

Treat it according to the above formulas for resolving *duàn cháng cǎo*. It is equally effective to drink *gān cǎo* water or *Dì Jiāng* (Earth Slurry).

解鹽滷毒 *Jiě Yán Lǔ Dú*
Resolving Bittern Poisoning[35]

生豆腐漿，冷服二三碗，至妙；如一時難得，以黃豆擂碎，沖冷水去渣服之 。

The patient should take two or three bowls of fresh cold soy milk. This is extremely wonderful. If it is difficult to obtain within an hour,[36] use soy beans

---

33. Today this herb is more commonly known as 雷公藤 *léi gōng téng*.
34. 野草 *yě cǎo* simply means weed. It is not clear if the author meant a specific plant.
35. Perhaps this means a more general salt toxicity which can occur when water intake is limited and excessive salt is consumed.
36. It is not clear if this refers to a Western single-hour or a Chinese double-

smashed into pieces. Drench them in cold water, remove the sediment, and have him drink it.

又方：白沙糖五六兩，用冷水調服，亦極效驗。

Another formula: The patient should take five or six *liǎng* of white granulated sugar mixed with cold water. This is also extremely effective and has been tested.

又方：淘米水冷服三四碗，亦可。

Another formula: He can also drink three or four bowls of cold water in which rice has been washed.

解鹼水毒 *Jiě Jiǎn Shuǐ Dú*
Resolving Lye Poisoning

照上解鹽滷毒各方治之。

Treat it according to the above formulas to resolve *Yán Lǔ* (bittern) poisoning.

解煤火毒 *Jiě Méi Huǒ Dú*
Resolving Coal or Charcoal Fire[37] Poisoning

中煤炭毒，土坑漏火氣而臭穢者，人受薰蒸，不覺自斃，其屍極輭，與夜臥夢魘不能復覺者相似。房中置水一盆，並使牕戶有透氣處，則煤炭雖臭，不能為害，飲冷水可解。或蘿蔔搗汁灌口鼻，移向風吹便醒。

People suffocate when struck by coal or charcoal toxins from an earthen *kàng*[38]

---

hour.

37. Carbon monoxide.

38. 土坑 *tǔ kàng* (earthen *kàng*): This is a traditional type of bed in the colder regions of China. It is a hollow platform made of brick or clay. Exhaust from a wood or coal stove is channeled through it to keep the sleeping people warm.

leaking fire qì with a foul odor. They are unaware that they are destroying themselves. The corpses are extremely soft, and it is similar to inability to wake up from oppressive ghost dreams during sleep at night. Place a basin of water in the room; at the same time ventilate the place through the windows and doors. Then it cannot cause harm, even if the coal or charcoal still smells bad. Drinking cold water can resolve it. Some crush radish to extract the juice and pour it into the mouth and nose. The victims will wake up when you move them into the blowing wind.

解迷悶藥 *Jiě Mí Mèn Yào*
Resolving Soporific Medicines[39]

飲涼水即解；重則飲藍靛汁立愈；如牙關緊閉，由鼻灌之，亦可 。

This will immediately resolve when the patient drinks cold water. If it is serious, he will immediately recover after drinking *lán diàn* liquid. If there is lockjaw, you can pour it in through the nose instead.

又方：白沙糖調冷水服，更妙 。

Another formula: Orally give white granulated sugar mixed with cold water. This is even more wonderful.

解百藥毒 *Jiě Bǎi Yào Dú*
Resolving Toxins from the Hundred Herbs [or Medicines]

凡服藥過多，致生瘡毒，頭腫如斗，脣破流血；或心口脹悶，或肚腹撮痛者 。用小黑豆 、綠豆（ 各一升 ）煮濃汁，冷服，即解 。

If not properly ventilated, the occupants may be poisoned by carbon monoxide.

39. This would include sedatives, tranquilizers, and things that might put a person in a stupor.

Whenever someone takes too much medicine, sores with toxins are generated. The head swells up until it is the size of a *dòu*.[40] The lips break open and bleed. Some have distention and oppression in the pit of the stomach, while others have cramping pain in the abdomen. Boil *xiǎo hēi dòu* and *lǜ dòu* (one *shēng* of each) into a concentrated liquid and let it cool. It will resolve when the patient takes it.

又方：甘草熬膏，日服數次，解毒如神，雖泄瀉，亦無害也。

Another formula: Simmer *gān cǎo* into a syrup. The patient should take it several times a day. It resolves toxins like a miracle! Even if it gives the patient diarrhea, it is still harmless.

又方：糯米糖食之，即解。或食白沙糖亦可。

Another formula: The toxins will resolve after eating glutinous rice sugar. The patient can also eat white granulated sugar.

又方：如已氣絕，祇須心間溫煖者，用防風二錢，煎水冷服，即活。

Another formula: When there is already expiration of qì, the patient can recover as long as the heart region is still warm: boil two *qián* of *fáng fēng* in water, let it cool, and give it to him.

解巴豆毒 *Jiě Bā Dòu Dú*
Resolving *Bā Dòu* Poisoning[41]

口渴面赤，五心煩躁，泄痢不止者是；用黑豆（一升）煮汁冷飲，即解。

The patient has thirst, red face, vexation and agitation of the five hearts, and

---

40. A 斗 *dòu* is equivalent to ten *shēng*. It is sometimes translated as a peck, although this is not precise.

41. The next several entries are substances used in Chinese medicine. See the appendix on p. 184 for their Latin names.

incessant diarrhea. Boil black soybeans (one *shēng*), let it cool, and have the patient drink the liquid. It will then resolve.

又方：川黃連，煎水冷服，亦效 。

Another formula: Boil *chuān huáng lián* in water, let it cool, and have the patient take it. This is also effective.

解附子烏頭天雄毒 *Jiě Fù Zǐ Wū Tóu Tiān Xióng Dú*
Resolving *Fù Zǐ, Wū Tóu,* or *Tiān Xióng* Poisoning[42]

防風（ 二錢 ）煎水飲；或照前解百毒方治之 。

Boil *fáng fēng* (two *qián*) in water and have the patient drink it. Some treat it according to the earlier formula for resolving the hundred toxins [*Dì Jiāng* (Earth Slurry)].

解芫花毒 *Jiě Yuán Huā Dú*
Resolving *Yuán Huā* Poisoning

治法與上附子毒同 。

The treatment method is the same as the above for *fù zǐ* poisoning.

解木鱉毒 *Jiě Mù Biē Dú*
Resolving *Mù Biē* Poisoning

身發抖戰者是；急用好肉桂（ 二錢 ）煎服立愈；或用香油一盞，和白沙糖（ 一兩 ）灌之，亦可；或照前解百毒方治之 。

The patient shivers and shakes. Quickly boil good quality *ròu guì* (two *qián*) and give it to him orally. He will immediately recover. You can also pour in a small-cup of sesame oil blended with white granulated sugar (one *liǎng*). Some

---

42. All are different types of aconite.

treat it according to the above formula for resolving the hundred toxins [*Dì Jiāng* (Earth Slurry)].

解硃砂毒 *Jiě Zhū Shā Dú*
Resolving *Zhū Shā* Poisoning

藍靛、韭汁飲之，即解。

It will resolve when the patient drinks *lán diàn* and Chinese leek juice.

解冰片毒 *Jiě Bīng Piàn Dú*
Resolving *Bīng Piàn* Poisoning

服冰片過多，口渴心煩；飲地漿一碗，冷服，即解。

When someone takes too much *bīng piàn* internally, he has thirst and heart vexation. The patient should drink a bowl of cold *Dì Jiāng* (Earth Slurry), and it will resolve.

解水銀毒 *Jiě Shuǐ Yín Dú*
Resolving Mercury Poisoning

服水銀欲死者，用真川椒（數斤）炒熱，鋪蓆下，令患者脫衣蓋被睡之，過一夜；水銀即從毛孔中，鑽入花椒內矣。

For someone who has taken mercury and is almost dead, stir-fry genuine *chuān jiāo* (several *jīn*) until it is hot, and spread it under a mat. Have the patient remove his clothing, cover up with bedding, and sleep on it. After a night, the mercury will have entered into the *huā jiāo* from the pores.

解鉛粉毒 *Jiě Qiān Fěn Dú*
Resolving *Qiān Fěn* Poisoning

婦人因打胎而服鉛粉，生子癡呆，身體多發瘡毒；用活鴨血乘熱服之，極為神效。

Women take *qiān fěn* to induce an abortion. Because of this she may give birth to a feeble-minded child [if he survives]. The body breaks out with many toxic sores. Give the patient live duck blood while it is still hot. This is extremely miraculous.

又方：白沙糖三四兩，冷水調服；或用蘿蔔搗汁飲之，均極效驗。

Another formula: Give three or four *liǎng* of white granulated sugar mixed in cold water. Some beat radish and drink the juice. They are both extremely effective.

解輕粉毒 *Jiě Qīng Fěn Dú*
Resolving *Qīng Fěn* Poisoning

輕粉性最燥烈，楊梅等瘡，服此雖易收功，其毒竄入經絡；或口齒腫爛，或筋骨疼痛攣縮；久而潰爛，經年累月，甚至終身不愈，致成殘廢。

The nature of *qīng fěn* is most fiery. Although taking it internally helps close red bayberry sores[43] and the like, its toxins steal into the channels and network vessels. Some end up with a swollen mouth and rotten teeth, and some suffer aching pain and contraction of the sinews and bones that can fester for a long time. Year after year passes without recovery over the course of one's life, and eventually the person becomes crippled.

方用土茯苓（一兩）、苡米、銀花、防風、木通、白鮮皮（各一錢）、木瓜（錢半）、皂莢子（四分）。

---

43. This refers to syphilitic sores.

The formula uses:

tǔ fú líng	土茯苓	1 *liǎng*
yǐ mǐ	苡米	1 *qián*
jīn yín huā	金銀花	1 *qián*
fang fēng	防風	1 *qián*
mù tōng	木通	1 *qián*
bái xiān pí	白鮮皮	1 *qián*
mù guā	木瓜	1.5 *qián*
zào jiá zǐ	皂莢子	4 *fēn*

右煎服，日服三次。

Boil the above and have the patient take it internally, three times a day.

氣虛加頂上黨參（一錢）；血虛加當歸（七分）。忌食茶並
牛、羊、雞、鵝、魚肉、燒酒、麵食、辣椒及一切發物，並
謹戒房事半年。服至十日，漸次痊愈，功效異常。

For qì vacuity, add superior quality *dǎng shēn* (one *qián*). For blood vacuity, add *dāng guī* (seven *fēn*). Avoid drinking tea, as well as beef, mutton, chicken, goose, or fish, white distilled liquor, food made of wheat, hot pepper, and all stimulating foods. Equally avoid bedroom affairs for half a year. The patient should take this formula for ten days. He will gradually recover. Its efficacy is extraordinary.

又方：紅棗丸服之，最為神效。

Another formula: The patient should take *Hóng Zǎo Wán*[44] orally. It is the most divinely effective.

---

44. 紅棗丸 *Hóng Zǎo Wán*: is described in Volume 11 of《驗方新編》 *Yàn Fāng Xīn Biān*. It consists of three *jīn* of 紅棗 *hóng zǎo*. Boil it using 杉木 *shān mù* as firewood. When cooked, peel off the skin and remove the seeds. Grind the ash from the *shān mù* into a fine powder. Blend evenly with the *hóng zǎo* pulp and make it into pills the size of a marble. This treats red bayberry [syphilitic] infection and toxic sores all over the body, including those from taking *qīng fěn* and other types of minerals. This should be taken faithfully every day without interruption. After recovery, continue taking it for one to two months to sever the root. *Hóng zǎo* can resolve toxins from elixir minerals. *Shān mù* is special for expelling invasion of damp-heat.

解斑蝥毒 *Jiě Bān Máo Dú*
Resolving *Bān Máo* Poisoning

黑豆（ 一升 ）煮濃汁，冷服即解 。

Boil black soybeans (one *shēng*) into a concentrated liquid and let it cool. It will resolve after the patient takes it.

又方：涼水調六一散七錢，服二三次，必痛止而愈 。

Another formula: Mix cold water with seven *qián* of *Liù Yī Sàn*.[45] The patient should take it two or three times. The pain will stop and he will recover.

又方：玉簪花根，煎水，冷服，即解 。

Another formula: Boil *yù zān huā gēn* in water and let it cool. It will resolve when the patient takes it.

解硫磺毒 *Jiě Liú Huáng Dú*
Resolving *Liú Huáng* Poisoning

方內生羊血為解硫磺神藥，愈後須戒殺生，並戒食羊為要 。
用真烏梅肉（ 焙乾，一兩，烏梅有李子假充者，以家製為
真 ）、白沙糖（ 五錢 ），煎服 。

Inside a formula, fresh goat blood is a miraculous medicine to resolve *liú huáng* toxins. After recovery, it is important to avoid killing and avoid eating goat. Use one *liǎng* of genuine *wū méi* flesh (stone-baked until dry. Plum is sometimes sold as *wū méi*[46] so take home-grown *wū méi* as genuine) and white granulated sugar (five *qián*). Boil it and give it to the patient orally.

---

45. 六一散 *Liù Yī Sàn*: Powder together six parts of 滑石 *huá shí* and one part of 甘草 *gān cǎo*. This formula clears summer heat and disinhibits dampness. Take six to nine grams each time by swallowing it with a liquid, or wrap it in gauze and decoct it. Take it once or twice a day.

46. 烏梅 *wū méi* is a type of Japanese apricot, not plum.

又方：防己（二錢），煎水，冷服，即解。

Another formula: Boil *fáng jǐ* (two *qián*) in water and let it cool, then give it to the patient. It will then resolve.

解花椒毒 *Jiě Huā Jiāo Dú*
Resolving *Huā Jiāo* Poisoning

口吐白沫，身冷氣欲絕者是，照前解百毒方治之，即愈。

Spitting white foam from the mouth, cold body, and qì that is about to expire. The patient will recover if treated according to the above formula for resolving the hundred toxins [*Dì Jiāng* (Earth Slurry)].

解食桐油毒 *Jiě Shí Tóng Yóu Dú*
Resolving Toxins from Eating Tung Oil

急飲熱酒，即解。

This will resolve if the patient quickly drinks hot liquor.

又方：真干柿餅食之即解。

Another formula: The toxins will resolve after eating genuine dried persimmons.

又方：蓮蓬，煎水服，甚效。

Another formula: Taking *lián péng* boiled in water is extremely effective.

解食蛇毒 *Jiě Shí Shé Dú*
Resolving Venom from Eating Snake

煙油用冷水洗出二三碗，飲之，凡受蛇毒，飲之其味必甘，並不難飲，屢試如神。或蛇遺毒在食物內，亦效。

Use two or three bowls of cold water to wash tobacco tar out [of a pipe] and have the patient drink [the wash water]. Whenever someone who is suffering from snake venom drinks this, it tastes sweet and is not difficult to drink. This has been repeatedly tried and works like a miracle! This is also effective when snakes leave venom behind inside the food.[47]

又方：蜈蚣一條，焙枯研末，冷水調服，一服即解 。如恐蜈蚣有毒，或一二日後照後解蜈蚣毒各方治之，決無後患 。

Another formula: Roast one *wú gōng* until dried out, powder it, mix with cold water, and take it. The toxins will resolve after one dose. If worried that the *wú gōng* has toxins, perhaps one or two days later, treat it according to the formula below on resolving *wú gōng* toxins. There will definitely be no more suffering.

解蜈蚣毒 *Jiě Wú Gōng Dú*
Resolving Centipede (*Wú Gōng*) Poisoning

凡誤食蜈蚣毒者，用樟樹葉，煎水冷服，極效 。

Whenever someone accidentally consumes centipede toxins, boil *zhāng shù yè* in water, let it cool, and give it to the patient. This is extremely effective.

又方：十指甲磨冷水，多飲之，其效無比 。

Another formula: Grind ten fingernails in cold water. Have the patient drink a large amount. The effect is incomparable.

又方：照前地漿方治之，均效 。

Another formula: It is equally effective to treat it according to the earlier formulas for *Dì Jiāng* (Earth Slurry).

---

47. Below we see that "田澗山溪，往往有蛇遺毒在內 。Snakes often leave venom behind in field gullies or mountain streams." So in this entry, we find it is possible to be poisoned by eating food in which a snake has left its venom, as well as from eating the poisonous snake itself.

蜈蚣入腹 *Wú Gōng Rù Fù*
A Centipede Enters the Abdomen

食生雞蛋二三個，略過半刻，再飲生油一盃，即吐出，絕
妙。

Have the patient eat two or three fresh chicken eggs. Wait for half a quarter hour.[48] Have him drink a cup of unrefined oil and then he will vomit it out. This is extremely clever.

解沙蟲水毒 *Jiě Shā Chóng Shuǐ Dú*
Resolving Sand Worm Water Toxins

萵苣菜搗汁，飲之，即解。

Crush *wō jù cài* to extract the juice and have the patient drink it. The toxins will then resolve.

又方：照前解百毒方治之。

Another formula: Treat it according to the above formula to resolve the hundred toxins [*Dì Jiāng* (Earth Slurry)].

解螞蝗毒 *Jiě Mǎ Huáng Dú*
Resolving Leech Toxins

（又名水蛭）此物入腹，久必生子，食人肝血，腹痛不可
忍，面目黃瘦，不治必死。用桂圓肉（荔枝肉亦可）包煙油
吞之，即死，隨於大便而出，屢試如神，此經驗第一方也。

This is also called *shuǐ zhì*. This thing goes into the abdomen and after a long time, it bears offspring. It feeds on human liver blood, which causes unendur-

---

48. It is not clear if this refers to half of a quarter Western single-hour (which would be 7.5 minutes) or half of a quarter Chinese double-hour (fifteen minutes).

able abdominal pain and a yellow thin face and eyes. If untreated, the patient will die. Wrap *guì yuán ròu* (*lì zhī ròu* is also usable) around tobacco tar and have the patient swallow it. The leeches will then die and will come out with the next bowel movement. It has been tried repeatedly and works like a miracle! This is the first choice for a formula based on experience.

又方：用白蜜頻頻食之，至一二斤，方愈。螞蟥火燒為末，見水即活，惟以蜜浸之，即化為水，故服蜜最佳。以多為妙，少則不效；如食蜜不愈，即食羊肉可化。白蜜，體虛不可多服，不如第一方之妙。

Another formula: The patient will recover when he repeatedly eats up to one or two *jīn* of white honey.[49] Fire burns leeches into a powder but if the leech is exposed to water it will revive. You can only soak it with honey; it will then dissolve and turn into water, so taking honey is the best. Using a lot is wonderful; using a small amount is not effective. If the patient eats honey but does not recover, he should eat mutton to dissolve the leech. Someone whose body is vacuous cannot take a lot of white honey so this is not as wonderful as the first formula.

又方：田中泥（ 一兩 ）、雄黃（ 二錢 ），右為丸，分作四服，開水下。其蟲入泥，隨大便而出。有時螞蟥行至鼻孔，血流不止；用田泥泡水一碗，放鼻孔前，必然乘泥而下。

Another formula: Make pills out of mud from the center of a field (*tián zhōng ní*, one *liǎng*) and *xióng huáng* (two *qián*), and divide it into four doses. Have the patient swallow it with boiled water. The leeches will go into the mud and will come out with the next bowel movement. Sometimes the leeches go into the nostrils, causing incessant bleeding. [In this case] soak field mud in a bowl of water and put the bowl in the front of the patient's nostrils; the leeches will inevitably take advantage of the mud and come out.

又方：青靛調水飲，即瀉出。

Another formula: Have the patient drink *qīng diàn* mixed with water. The leeches will go out with diarrhea.

---

49. White honey means good quality honey.

又方：蘆藜炒為末，調服一錢，必吐出。

Another formula: Stir-fry and powder *lú lí*. Mix it [with a liquid] and have the patient take one *qián*. He will vomit the leeches out.

解河豚魚毒 *Jiĕ Hé Tún Yú Dú*
Resolving Globefish (*Hé Tún*) Poisoning

槐花（微炒）與乾胭脂等分，同搗成粉，冷水調服，極效。

Pound equal portions of *huái huā* (slightly stir-fried) and *gān yān zhī* (rouge) together into a powder. Mix it with cold water and have the patient take it internally. It is extremely effective.

又方：多食橄欖；並用橄欖核磨水服，極效。

Another formula: Have the patient eat a lot of *gǎn lǎn*.[50] At the same time grind *gǎn lǎn hé* and have the patient take it internally with water. This is extremely effective.

又方：照前解百毒方治之。

Another formula: Treat it according to the above formula for resolving the hundred toxins [*Dì Jiāng* (Earth Slurry)].

解各色魚毒 *Jiĕ Gè Sè Yú Dú*
Resolving Every Kind of Fish Poisoning

紫蘇煎濃汁，冷服極效，以多為妙。

Boil *zǐ sū* [*yè*] into a concentrated liquid and let it cool. Taking this is extremely effective, and using a lot is wonderful.

---

50. 橄欖 *gǎn lǎn* (Canarii alba) is Chinese 'olive.' It is not the same as the Mediterranean olive. *Gǎn lǎn* grows in Southern China. The dried fruit and nuts are eaten. The fresh fruit may be used in stir-fried dishes.

又方：多食橄欖，並用橄欖核磨水服，最效 。

Another formula: Have the patient eat a lot of *gǎn lǎn*. At the same time grind *gǎn lǎn hé* and have the patient take it internally with water. This is the most effective.

又方：食魚過多，腹脹面黃者，用紅麴（ 三合 ）煮爛，連渣服，即從大便出，連服三次愈 。

Another formula: For someone who has eaten too much fish, with a distended abdomen and yellow face, boil *hóng qū* (three *gě*) until soft. Have the patient take it, including the dregs, and the poison will then come out with his bowel movement. Recovery comes after taking it three consecutive times.

解食鱉毒 *Jiě Shí Biē Dú*
Resolving Toxins from Eating Soft-Shelled Turtle

飲藍靛汁，即解 。

It will resolve after drinking *lán diàn* liquid.

又方：冷水調鹽飲之，效 。

Another formula: Drinking cold water mixed with salt is effective.

又方：淡豆豉（ 一合 ）搗爛，冷水沖入，取汁服，即愈 。

Another formula: Pound *dàn dòu chǐ* (one *gě*) to a pulp, and drench it in cold water. Recovery will come after taking the juice internally.

解蝦蟆毒 *Jiě Há Má Dú*
Resolving Toad Toxins

照上鱉毒各方治之，即解 。

It will resolve after treating it according to the different formulas above for soft-shelled turtle (*biē*) toxins.

解黃白鱔毒 *Jiě Huáng Bái Shàn Dú*
Resolving Yellow Eel and White Eel Toxins

照上鼈毒各方治之。

Treat it according to the different formulas above for soft-shelled turtle (*biē*) toxins.

解螃蟹毒 *Jiě Páng Xiè Dú*
Resolving Crab Poisoning

紫蘇煎濃汁，冷服二三碗，即解。生藕汁、生大蒜汁、生冬瓜汁、生黑豆汁，俱可解。

Boil *zǐ sū* [*yè*] into a concentrated liquid, and let it cool. The poisoning will resolve when the patient takes two or three bowls of it. The following can resolve crab poisoning: fresh lotus root juice, fresh garlic juice, fresh winter melon juice, and fresh black soybean liquid.

解犬馬肉毒 *Jiě Quǎn Mǎ Ròu Dú*
Resolving Dog and Horse Meat Poisoning

凡食犬肉，腹脹口渴，發熱亂言者，用淡豆豉（二兩）、杏仁（三兩），同蒸搗爛，服之，日服二三次；或煮蘆茅根飲之，俱效。

If there is abdominal distention, thirst, fever, and raving following the consumption of dog meat, steam *dàn dòu chǐ* (two *liǎng*) and *xìng rén* (three *liǎng*) together, and then pound them into a pulp. Have the patient take it two or three times a day. Some boil *lú máo gēn* and have the patient drink it. Both are effective.

又方：杏仁（二兩，去皮）蒸熟，研爛，用滾水和勻，取汁服；服後必泄，俟泄三次後，再服冷醋一茶鍾。或冷粥一碗，即愈。

Another formula: Steam *xìng rén* (two *liǎng*, remove the skin) until hot and grind it into a pulp. Blend it evenly with boiling water and have the patient take the liquid. Diarrhea will follow. After after three bouts of diarrhea, give the patient a tea cup of cold vinegar. Others have the patient eat a bowl of cold rice congee. He will then recover.

又方：荸薺皮（焙枯，研末，三分）、紫背浮萍（焙枯，研末，三分），共和勻，開水調服，即腹響如雷，大吐大泄而愈；各種食積腹脹如鼓者，服之皆效。

Another formula: Blend *bí qí pí* (stone-baked until dry and ground into a powder, three *fēn*) and *zǐ bèi fú píng* (stone-baked until dry and ground into a powder, three *fēn*) together evenly. Mix this with boiled water and have the patient take it. The patient will recover when there are thunderous abdominal sounds, great vomiting, and great diarrhea. Taking this is effective for different types of food accumulation with drum-like abdominal distention.

解食牛肉毒 *Jiě Shí Niú Ròu Dú*
Resolving Toxins from Eating Beef

苦瓜皮，搗爛沖水服，神效。

It is miraculously effective to pound the peel of bitter melon until soft, drench it in water, and take it.

又方：菊花連根搗汁酒服，均效。

Another formula: Pound *jú huā* including the roots to make juice and take it with liquor. This is equally effective.

又方：人乳，飲之即解。

Another formula: The toxins will resolve after drinking human milk.

解鵝鴨毒 *Jiě É Yā Dú*
Resolving Toxins from [Eating] Goose and Duck

糯米半斤，淘水去米，溫服一碗即愈 。

Wash a half *jīn* of polished glutinous rice in water and remove the rice. The patient will recover when he takes a bowl of this water that has been warmed.

解雞肉毒 *Jiě Jī Ròu Dú*
Resolving Toxins from [Eating] Chicken

地漿飲之可解 。

It can resolve after drinking *Dì Jiāng* (Earth Slurry).

解馬肉毒 *Jiě Mǎ Ròu Dú*
Resolving Horse Meat Poisoning

人乳飲之即解，或照前解百毒方治之 。

Have the patient drink human milk for recovery. Some treat it according to the above formula for resolving the hundred toxins [*Dì Jiāng* (Earth Slurry)].

解鬱肉漏脯毒 *Jiě Yù Ròu Lòu Pú Dú*
Resolving *Yù Ròu* and *Lòu Pú* Poisoning[51]

凡各肉密器緊蓋過夜者，為鬱肉；屋漏沾著者，為漏脯；皆有毒 。韭菜搗汁飲之，即解 。

Whenever any meat that is enclosed in a tightly covered container is left out overnight, it is called *yù ròu*. *Lòu pú* occurs when a leak in the roof moistens

---

51. These terms are difficult to translate. 鬱肉 *yù ròu* is something like 'stagnant meat.' 漏脯 *lòu pú* could be translated as 'leaky meat.' The entry belows explain what these items actually are.

this meat. They both have toxins. The patient will recover when you crush *jiŭ cài* to extract the juice and have him drink it.

解諸肝毒 *Jiě Zhū Gān Dú*
Resolving All Liver Toxins

照前解百毒方地漿飲之，極效 。

Drink *Dì Jiāng* (Earth Slurry) according to the above formula for resolving the hundred toxins.

又方：熟豬油（ 一斤 ）拌飯，或炒飯，亦可 。分作一二日食盡，此一二日內，勿食別物為要 。

Another formula: Cooked pork lard (one *jīn*) mixed with cooked rice. It can also be stir-fried with rice. Divide it into portions for one or two days and have the patient eat it all. It is very important that during these one or two days, he does not eat anything else.

解自死各物毒 *Jiě Zì Sǐ Gè Wù Dú*
Resolving Various Toxins from Eating Things that have Died on their Own

黃柏研末，冷水調，服一二錢，即解 。或飲人乳一碗，極效 。

Grind *huáng bǎi* into a powder, and mix it with cold water. Have the patient take one or two *qián* to resolve it, or drink a bowl of human milk. This is extremely effective.

解藥箭射傷鳥獸肉毒
Jiě Yào Jiàn Shè Shāng Niǎo Shòu Ròu Dú
Resolving Toxins from Eating the Meat of Birds and Beasts that have been Shot by a Poison Arrow

先以鹽水服之，次以黑豆煮濃汁飲之，即解。

First have the patient take salt water internally. Next he should drink the concentrated liquid of boiled black soybeans, and this will resolve it.

又方：蘆茅根煮熟，連湯食，極效。

Another formula: Boil *lú máo gēn* thoroughly, and have the patient eat it along with the broth. This is extremely effective.

又方：照前解百毒方治之，更妙。

Another formula: Even more wonderful, treat it according to the above formula for resolving the hundred toxins [*Dì Jiāng* (Earth Slurry)].

解杏仁毒 *Jiě Xìng Rén Dú*
Resolving *Xìng Rén* Poisoning

杏仁生、熟飲之，均不為害，若火炒不透，半生半熟者，服十數粒，即死；其屍眼閉，舌唇耳竅手足十指俱青色，腹有青塊，惟急吐可解。用杏樹皮煎湯飲之，雖迷亂將死，亦可救。或用麝香（一分）沖水服。

Drinking fresh or cooked *xìng rén* does no harm. But if the fire of stir-frying does not penetrate all the way and it is half fresh and half cooked – when someone takes ten or more pieces, he will die. The eyes of the corpse will be closed. The orifices of the tongue, lips, and ears, as well as the ten fingers and toes will all be green-blue (*qīng*), and there will be green-blue lumps in the abdomen. This can only be resolved by quick vomiting. Boil *xìng shù pí* and have the patient drink the broth. Even if he is dazed and about to die, he can still be rescued. Some drench *shè xiāng* (one *fēn*) in water and have him take it.

解百果毒 *Jiě Bǎi Guǒ Dú*
Resolving Poisoning from the Hundred Fruits

麝香（一分），煎湯服，即解。

This will resolve when you boil *shè xiāng* (one *fēn*) and have the patient drink the decoction.

解木瓜毒 *Jiě Mù Guā Dú*
Resolving *Mù Guā* Poisoning

舌大滿口者是，用好醋調黃糖（紅糖亦可）含口中，吐出涎水數次，即愈。

The tongue grows large and fills the mouth. Mix good quality vinegar with yellow sugar (red sugar can also be used)[52] and have the patient hold it inside his mouth. He will recover after spitting out saliva several times.

解豆腐毒 *Jiě Dòu Fǔ Dú*
Resolving Tofu Poisoning

蘿蔔煎湯飲之，即解。

This will resolve when the patient drinks soup of boiled radish.

解飲田澗山溪水毒 *Jiě Yǐn Tián Jiàn Shān Xī Shuǐ Dú*
Resolving Toxins from Drinking Water of
Field Gullies and Mountain Streams

凡田澗山溪，往往有蛇遺毒在內；如誤飲其水，用水調雄黃，多服數次，自愈。

---

52. 黃糖 *huáng táng* is literally yellow sugar, but it is what we might call light brown sugar. 紅糖 *hóng táng* translates literally as red sugar and is equivalent to our brown sugar.

Snakes can frequently leave venom behind in field gullies or mountain streams. If someone accidentally drinks this water, mix water with *xióng huáng* and have him drink a large amount several times. He will automatically recover.

解隔夜茶水毒 *Jiě Gé Yè Chá Shuǐ Dú*
Resolving Poisoning from the Previous Night's Tea

服雄黃或地漿，均可解。

Have the patient take *xióng huáng* or *Dì Jiāng* (Earth Slurry). They can equally resolve the poison.

諸毒須知 *Zhū Dú Xū Zhī*
What Should Be Known About Various Toxins

久閉空房毒：凡屋宇久閉，陰濕閉結不散，或邪魅借以潛蹤，蛇虺惡獸從而盤踞，宜大張聲勢，或先以火驚散。

Toxins from a house that has been closed up for a long time: Whenever a house is closed up for a long time, yīn dampness is closed in, binds up, and does not disperse. Sometimes evil demons borrow the house in order to hide out; venomous snakes and fierce beasts follow and entrench themselves. It is suitable to put on a big event with lots of noise or first frighten the evil things away with fire.

山洞園林毒：凡偏僻山洞及年久園亭、藤蘿、花樹之下，不可飲食，恐有蛇虺毒蟲游行其上，遺毒於食物中，為害不小。

Toxins from a mountain cave or forest park: Do not eat or drink when in remote mountain caves or under aging garden pavilions, Chinese wisteria (*téng luó*), flowers, and trees. There is the risk of venomous snakes and toxic *chóng*[53] up above leaving toxins in the food; the harm it causes is not small.

---

53. 蟲 *chóng*: A reminder here that *chóng* can mean various types of creep-crawly things, not just bugs and worms.

衣有暑毒：夏日汗透之衣，向日中晒晾，忽豪雨將至，急為收檢，則烈日之毒即蘊於內，如遇酷暑汗出時，偶一衣之，則暑以引暑，立中其毒。又夏秋晒晾冬衣，必須冷透收檢。若未攤冷而收入箱籨，將來穿著必受暑毒。宜於臨穿先一時、當風吹透再穿，方免其害。

Summerheat-toxins in the clothes: Sweat can soak the clothes on a summer day while roasting in the sun around noontime, or a sudden torrential rain may arrive. Toxins from the scorching sun are contained inside the clothes when they are quickly gathered up and put away. Then if by chance these same clothes are worn during a time of intense summerheat, there will be an immediate summerheat stroke because summerheat attracts summerheat. In addition, when wearing clothes in the winter that roasted in the sun during summer and autumn, the cold penetrates into the clothes when they are gathered up and put away. If the cold is not [dispersed by] spreading out the clothes before storing then in a chest, summerheat toxins will be received when they are worn in the future. Wait an hour before wearing the clothes and first let the wind blow through them; the harm can be avoided in this way.

草藥毒：山有毒草，入山采藥，須細心揀淨。

Herbal medicine toxins: There are toxic herbs in the mountains. When picking herbs in the mountains, be careful to select the clean ones.

隔夜茶水食物毒：凡夜間茶水、食物未經蓋好，必有蟲、鼠遺毒，不可誤飲。

Toxins from tea or food left out overnight: Whenever tea or food is not well covered at night, it will have toxins left by *chóng* and rats. Do not eat it by mistake.

雞毒：雞食蜈蚣、百蟲久，則食之傷人。故養生家，雞老不食。又，夏不食雞。

Toxins from chicken: It is harmful to eat a chicken that has eaten *wú gōng* or the hundred *chóng* for a long time. So masters of nourishing life do not eat old chickens. They also do not eat chicken in the summer.

屋漏水毒：屋漏滴食物上，食之有毒。

Toxins due to water from a leaky roof: If a leaky roof drips onto food, there are toxins when it is eaten.

諸果有異樣者，根下必有毒蛇。果未成核者、食之發癰瘡，並發寒熱。果落地有蟲緣過者，食之生痔漏。有雙蒂者，有雙子者，有沉水者，均有毒，不可食。

All fruits that have peculiarities – there must be venomous snakes at the roots of the tree. Eating a fruit that does not make a pit will make abscesses and sores erupt, as well as fever and sensations of cold. Fruits that fall to the ground have *chóng* because they are over-ripe; eating them engenders hemorrhoids and fistulas. Fruits with double stems or double seeds, or that sink in water are all equally toxic and cannot be eaten.

Chapter 3

误吞諸物 *Wù Tūn Zhū Wù*
Accidentally Swallowing Various Things

Translator's Note: This chapter is abridged from Volume 12 of 《驗方新編》*Yàn Fāng Xīn Biān*.

误吞鐵器 *Wù Tūn Tiě Qì*
Accidentally Swallowing Ironware

炭皮研末，調粥二三碗，食之。炭末即裹鐵器，由大便而出，神效。

Grind *tàn pí*[54] into a powder, mix it into two or three bowlfuls of congee and have the patient eat it. Charcoal powder immediately binds to ironware, and the object will come out in the stool. This has miraculous effects.

误吞鐵鍼 *Wù Tūn Tiě Zhēn*
Accidentally Swallowing an Iron Needle

蠶豆煮韭菜同食，鍼與菜從大便而出（無蠶豆，用鹽蛋亦可）。

Boil *cán dòu* and *jiǔ cài* together and have the patient eat it. The needle will

---

54. 炭皮 *tàn pí* or 木炭皮 *mù tàn pí* is a thin 'skin' on the outside of a piece of charcoal. It can be peeled off and seems to have a different function from the whole piece or the core of the charcoal.

come out in the stool with the leeks. (If you don't have *cán dòu*, you can substitute salted eggs.)

又方：照前木炭皮研末，和粥食之，亦出。

Another formula: Grind *mù tàn pí* into powder, blend with congee, and have the patient eat it, as described in the previous entry. This will also make the needle come out.

誤吞金銀銅鐵錫鉛 *Wù Tūn Jīn Yín Tóng Tiě Xī Qiān*
Accidentally Swallowing Gold, Silver, Copper, Iron, Tin, or Lead

羊脛骨（即羊前腿膝蓋骨也），燒枯為末，米湯調服二三錢，一日必出。

Roast sheep [or goat] shin bone (*yáng jìng gǔ*, meaning the knee cap[55] of a sheep's front leg) until dried out and powder it. Mix it with rice soup and give the patient two or three *qián*. The object will come out in one day.

又方：橄欖核燒枯，研末，開水調服，自出。

Another formula: Roast *gǎn lǎn hé* until dried out, then grind them into a powder. Mix with boiled water and have the patient take it internally. The object will automatically come out.

又方：糯米糖，食半斤，亦效。

Another formula: Eat half a *jīn* of glutinous rice sugar. This is also effective.

又方：韭菜一把，滾水煮軟，不切斷，淡食之，少頃，即吐出，或從大便而出。

Another formula: Cook a handful of *jiǔ cài* in boiling water until soft, but do not cut them. Have the patient eat them bland [unsalted]. In a short while, he will vomit the object out, or sometimes it comes out with the stool.

---

55. Translator's note: This doesn't make sense. The shin bone or tibia is not the knee cap or patella.

誤吞金箔 *Wù Tūn Jīn Bó*
Accidentally Swallowing Gold Leaf

此物吞下，或閉喉管，或閉肺管，遲則難救。急取羊血灌之，最為神效。

When this is swallowed, it sometime blocks the esophagus or the bronchial tubes. If you hesitate, it is difficult to save the patient. Quickly pour sheep [or goat] blood into him. This has extremely miraculous effects.

誤吞銅錢 *Wù Tūn Tóng Qián*
Accidentally Swallowing Copper Coins

多食荸薺，自然消化，其效無比。

Eat a lot of water chestnuts (*bí qí*). The coins will naturally be digested. The effect is incomparable.

又方：砂仁（ 二兩 ），煎湯服之，亦化。或照上誤吞金銀等方治之，亦可。

Another formula: Decoct *shā rén* (two *liǎng*) and have the patient take it. This also dissolves the coins. This can also be treated according to the above formulas for accidentally swallowing gold, silver, etc.

諸骨卡喉 *Zhū Gú Kǎ Hóu*
Various Types of Bones Stuck in the Throat

此症宜急治之，若飲食難進，餓倒胃氣，殊屬難救。

This condition must be treated quickly; if it is difficult for the person to drink and eat, stomach qì will collapse from starvation. It is especially difficult to save such a person.

又方：有人被魚骨橫梗胸中，半月不下，疼痛叫喚，用橄欖核磨濃汁，滾水調服，即愈。真仙方也。

Another formula: Sometimes a fish bone gets stuck horizontally in someone's chest and cannot go down for half a month; it is so painful that they cry out. Grind *gǎn lǎn hé* and make a concentrated liquid. Mix it with boiling water. The patient will recover after taking it. This is a true formula of the immortals.

又方：灰麵（四兩），用冷水調稠，敷兩膝頭上，約一時久，其骨即化，真奇方也，一切禽魚獸骨，皆治。

Another formula: Mix *huī miàn*[56] (four *liǎng*) with cold water until it is thick, and apply it to both knee caps. After about an hour,[57] the bone will dissolve. This formula is truly extraordinary. It treats all types of bird, fish, or animal bones.

又方：真南硼砂取一塊含之，即愈。

Another formula: The patient will recover after sucking on a lump of genuine *nán péng shā*.[58]

又方：有人因一骨梗喉，百藥不下，夢人告之服真南硼砂（黃色如膠者真）最妙。

Another formula: There was a person who had a bone stuck in his throat and the hundred herbal medicines did not make it go down. In a dream, someone told him to take genuine *nán péng shā* (the genuine is yellow and glue-like). This is most wonderful!

又方：食山查膏，甚效。或以山查煎濃汁，服之，亦可。緣雞骨入山查膏即化，故能治一切骨梗也。

---

56. 灰麵 *huī miàn*, literally 'grey flour,' is flour that is mixed with the juice of herbs, including 蓬柴草 *péng chái cáo*, also known as 白莖鹽生草 *bái jīng yán shēng cǎo* (Halogoton arachnoideus). This turns it grey, hence its name.

57. It is not clear if this refers to a Western single-hour or a Chinese double-hour.

58. 南硼砂 *nán péng shā* and 硼砂 *péng shā* both refer to borax. However, in the next item we find that *nán péng shā* is yellow and glue-like.

Another formula: Eating *shān zhá* paste[59] is extremely effective. *Shān zhá* can also be boiled into a concentrated liquid and have the patient take it internally. The reason this works is that chicken bones dissolve when they absorb the *shān zhá* paste. Therefore it is able to treat all bones stuck in the throat.

又方：貫眾（ 焙枯研末 ），每服一二錢，神效 。或煎濃湯，含口中，緩緩嚥下，亦可 。

Another formula: Each dose is one or two *qián* of *guàn zhòng* (stone-baked until dry, then powdered). This has miraculous effects. It can also be boiled into a concentrated decoction and held in the mouth, swallowing it little by little.

又方：大蒜塞鼻不令透氣，其骨自下 。

Another formula: Stop up the nose with garlic so that qí (air) cannot penetrate through it. The bone will automatically descend.

又方：白糖含口中令其自消，則骨與之俱化矣 。

Another formula: Hold white sugar in the mouth and let it spontaneously dissolve; the bone will completely melt along with the sugar.

又方：魚骨卡者，以本魚骨插耳尖縫內，左卡插左，右卡插右，神效 。

Another formula: When a fish bone is stuck in the throat, use a bone from the same fish and stick it inside the crevice of the ear apex. If the bone is stuck on the left side, stick it in the left ear; if it is stuck on the right, stick it in the right ear. This is miraculously effective.

又方：栗子內薄皮，瓦上焙枯存性研末，吹入喉中即下 。

Another formula: Roast the inner thin skin of chestnuts on a tile until it is dry, preserving its nature, grind it into a powder, and blow it into the throat. The bone will go down.

---

59. *Shān zhá* paste is basically made the same way as applesauce, except *shān zhá* is used instead of apples.

又方：砂仁、草果、威靈仙（ 各三錢 ）。加白糖（ 一兩 ），
水煎，連服三四碗。無論何骨俱化，神效。

Another formula: *Shā rén, cǎo guǒ,* and *wēi líng xiān* (three *qián* of each). Add white sugar, (one *liǎng*) and boil it in water, then have the patient drink three or four bowls, one after the other. It doesn't matter which type of bone was swallowed, as they will all be dissolved. This has miraculous effects.

又方：製燈心炭，研極細，吹入三四吹，神效。

Another formula: Make charcoal of *dēng xīn*, and grind it into an extremely fine powder. Blow it into the throat three or four times. This has miraculous effects.

又方：魚膽飲：冬天取鱖魚膽懸掛陰乾，遇有各骨卡喉，即
取一個（ 大者半個亦可 ），水煎溫服，少時嘔吐，骨即隨
出。如尚未吐，再服溫酒，以吐為度，酒隨量飲。若再未
出，再飲魚膽服之，無不出者。如各骨在腹內日久。刺疼黃
瘦者。服之皆出。草魚鯽魚膽。皆可。竹木卡喉者。服之亦
極效。

Another formula: *Yú Dǎn Yǐn* (Fish Gall Bladder Drink): In the wintertime hang the gall bladder from *guì yú*[60] in the shade to dry. If you come across any type of fishbone stuck in the throat, boil one gall bladder (or half a large one) in water and have the patient take it warm. A moment later he will vomit and the bone will come out. If he doesn't vomit, he should also take a dose of warm liquor. Use vomiting as the measure [of when to stop], giving the liquor according to the patient's capacity to drink. If it still doesn't come out, he should drink another dose of the fish gall bladder. There is never a case when the bone does not come out. If any bones are stuck inside the abdomen, there will be pricking pain, yellowing and emaciation over the course of time. All the bones will come out when he takes this formula. Both *cǎo yú*[61] and *jì yú*[62] gall bladder can be used. Taking it is also extremely effective for pieces of bamboo or wood stuck in the throat.

---

60. Mandarin fish (Sinipearcae Vesica Fellea).
61. Grass carp (Ctenopharyngodonis Caro).
62. Golden carp (Carassii Aurati).

又方：吳茱萸煎濃汁飲一碗。骨至腹中者，亦軟而易下。

Another formula: Boil *wú zhū yú* into a thick liquid and drink a bowl. Bones down to the abdomen will soften so it is easy for them to go down.

又方：五月五日午時，在韭菜地內面東勿語，取蚯蚓泥收之。每用少許擦喉外，其骨自消。

On the fifth day of the fifth lunar month, in a place where *jiǔ cài* grows, face east and do not speak. Collect earthworm mud. Each time, rub a little on the outside of the throat. The bone will automatically dissolve.

稻穀卡喉 *Dào Gǔ Kǎ Hóu*
Rice Husks Stuck in the Throat

紫花地丁，細嚼吞之，神效。

Have the patient take *zǐ huā dì dīng*. He should chew it carefully and swallow it. This has miraculous effects.

又方：食糯米糖亦下。

Another formula: The rice husks will also go down when the patient eats glutinous rice sugar.

竹木卡喉 *Zhú Mù Kǎ Hóu*
A Piece of Bamboo or Wood Stuck in the Throat

老絲瓜燒灰，每服三錢，兌酒下。

Reduce an old *sī guā* to ashes, and have the patient take three *qián* each dose. Add it to liquor and swallow it.

又方：照前骨卡喉魚膽飲方服之，極效。

Another formula: The patient should take the above formula *Yú Dǎn Yǐn* for treating bones stuck in the throat. This is extremely effective.

74

又方：木卡喉者，鐵斧磨水灌下，即愈，勿令人見。

Another formula: To recover from wood stuck in the throat, pour the water used in grinding an iron ax into the patient. Do not let the person see [what it is you are using].

又方：竹木卡喉者，製燈草炭，開水送下，即愈。外用燈草炭，放膏藥上，貼喉痛處，一夜即消。

Another formula: For someone with bamboo or wood stuck in his throat, make *dēng cǎo* charcoal. He will recover after swallowing it with boiled water. Externally, place *dēng cǎo* charcoal on a plaster and stick it onto the painful site on the throat. The bone will disperse overnight.

諸豆卡喉 *Zhū Dòu Kǎ Hóu*
Various Types of Beans Stuck in the Throat

土狗蟲數個（ 又名螻蛄 ），搗爛敷喉外腫處，其豆自下。

Pound several *tǔ gǒu chóng* into a pulp and apply them to the swollen site on the outside of the throat. The bean will automatically go down.

鐵鈎卡喉 *Tiě Gōu Kǎ Hóu*
An Iron Hook Stuck in the Throat

有童子誤吞釣鈎，將鈎線一扯，鈎已穿入喉管，片時頸如斗大，後用佛珠穿入鈎線，漸漸將珠挨進，直至喉管，輕輕將珠向內一推，其鈎已脫出在珠上，緊執珠繩抽出，即愈。

Sometimes a child accidentally swallows a fishhook. When he pulls on the hook line, the hook gets caught in the throat. In a moment, the neck swells to the size of a *dòu*.[63] String prayer beads onto the hook line, little by little letting the beads go in one by one until they fill the line down the esophagus. Lightly

---

63. A 斗 *dòu* is equivalent to ten *shēng*. It is sometimes translated as a peck, although this is not precise.

and gently give the beads a push inward. The hook will come off in the beads. Hold the bead cord tightly and draw it out. The patient will then recover.

頭髮卡喉 *Tóu Fà Kǎ Hóu*
Head Hair Stuck in the Throat

舊木梳燒枯為末，酒沖服 。

Roast an old wooden comb until it is dried out and powder it. Drench it in liquor and have the patient take it.

又方：亂髮（ 燒灰 ），水調一錢服 。髮灰須令燒盡；如有生髮未經燒者，食之害人 。

Another formula: Reduce hair[64] into ashes. Mix one *qián* with water and have the patient take it. The hair ash must be completely burnt; if there is fresh unburnt hair, eating it will harm the patient.

---

64. 亂髮 *luàn fà* (Crinis Crinis): According to Wiseman, this simply refers to hair. The term literally means 'chaotic hair.' The last chapter of this book says the hair is rolled up into a hard ball.

Chapter 4

煙酒醉傷 *Yān Jiǔ Zuì Shāng*
Damage from Smoking or Alcohol Intoxication

Translator's Note: This chapter is abridged from Volume 12 of 《驗方新編》 *Yàn Fāng Xīn Biān* where both this and the previous chapter come under the heading of Accidentally Swallowing Various Things.

水旱煙醉傷 *Shuǐ Hàn Yān Zuì Shāng*
Damage from Addiction to Smoking a Hookah or Pipe

胡黃連（ 一錢 ），煎水兌茶服，即解 。

Boil *hú huáng lián* (one *qián*) in water and add tea. The patient will recover when he takes it.

洋煙醉傷 *Yáng Yān Zuì Shāng*
Damage from Tobacco Addiction

飲鹽水即解，或飲醬油，或飲糖水，均效 。

This will resolve after drinking salt water, soy sauce, or sugar water. They are equally effective.

酒醉傷 *Jiǔ Zuì Shāng*
Damage from Alcohol Intoxication

凡酒醉死者，急解醉人頭髮，放新汲井水盆內，將衣解開，
用豆腐遍身貼之，（ 無豆腐，用布泡井水貼之 ），少刻再
換，換至數次必醒 。惟寒天不宜 。

Whenever someone is dead drunk, quickly resolve the drunkenness by putting
the person's head hair in a basin of newly drawn well water, undo his clothing,
and apply tofu on his entire body (if you do not have tofu, apply cloth soaked
in well water on him). Change it after a little while; he will sober up once you
have changed it several times. The only time this is not appropriate is in cold
weather.

樟樹子（ 四錢 ），酒三盃煎滾，候溫灌之，即醒 。或用樟木
（ 二兩 ），煎水服，亦可 。此仙方也，屢試如神 。如牙關緊
閉，用烏梅搽牙，以瓷調羹撬開灌下，或打開一牙灌入 。切
不可以身冷脈絕而不救也 。

Boil *zhāng shù zǐ* (four *qián*) in three wine-cups of liquor. Wait until it is warm
[not hot] and pour it in. The patient will then wake up. You can also boil *zhāng
mù* (two *qián*) in water and give it to him. This formula is from the immortals. It
has been repeatedly tested and works like a miracle. If the jaw is clenched shut,
rub *wū méi* into the teeth, force the jaw open with a porcelain spoon, and pour
the medicine down. Some break out a tooth to pour it in. Be sure to attempt to
rescue someone even when the body is cold and the pulse is expiring.

又方：麝香（ 半分 ），放口中，即醒 。

Another formula: Place *shè xiāng* (a half *fēn*) in the patient's mouth. He will
then wake up.

又方：黑豆（ 一升 ），煮汁，乘溫灌下三盞，即醒 。

Another formula: Boil black soybeans (one *shēng*) for the liquid. Take advantage of its warmth and pour down three small-cups. He will then wake up.

又方：白蘿卜汁，或熱尿灌之，俱效。

Another formula: Pour white radish juice or hot urine into him. They are both effective.

酒醉心痛 *Jiǔ Zuì Xīn Tòng*
Heart Pain from Alcohol Intoxication[65]

白沙糖（ 三、四兩 ），淡酒沖服，止痛如神。

Drench white granulated sugar (three or four *liǎng*) in weak liquor and give it to the patient. It stops pain like a miracle!

酒醉小便不通 *Jiǔ Zuì Xiǎo Biàn Bù Tōng*
Inhibited Urination from Alcohol Intoxication

葛花（ 三錢 ）、燈芯（ 七根 ），右酒煮服，即通。

Boil *gé huā* (three *qián*) and *dēng xīn* (seven strands) in liquor and give it to the patient. Urine will then pass.

酒病大小便不通 *Jiǔ Bìng Dà Xiǎo Biàn Bù Tōng*
Inhibited Defecation and Urination from Liquor Disease

生薑汁（ 一茶鍾 ）、黃蠟（ 一錢 ）、白礬（ 五分 ）右共煎滾，加燒酒一碗，沖入飲之，立能止痛。再用藤菜煎水，燻前後陰，大小便即通。百藥不效者，此方用之如神。忌食雞肉十日。

Boil *shēng jiāng* juice (one tea cup), beeswax (one *qián*), and *bái fán* (five *fēn*) together, then add a bowl of white distilled liquor and drink it. It can immediately stop the pain. Next boil *téng cài* in water to steam the anterior and posterior yīn. Stool and urine will then pass. The hundred medicines are not

---

65. This may refer to true heart pain or epigastric pain. It is probably the latter.

effective but this formula works like a miracle! The patient should avoid eating chicken for ten days.

酒病 *Jiǔ Bìng*
Liquor Disease

好飲之人，酒毒發作，頭痛目眩，或咽喉閉悶。或下痢清水，日數十次，形神痿頓。

People who like to drink show the effects of liquor toxins, with headache and dizzy vision, or blockage and oppression of the throat. Some have clear water diarrhea, more than ten times a day. The body atrophies and the spirit is ruined.

宜用陳皮（五錢）、甘草（二錢）、川連（三錢），右三味，俱微炒為末，再配松花粉（一兩），和勻。每服二錢，早晚以開水送下一服，兩日即愈。

You should use *chén pí* (five *qián*), *gān cǎo* (two *qián*), and *chuān lián* (three *qián*). Lightly stir-fry the above three medicinals and powder them. Then add *sōng huā fěn* (one *liǎng*) and blend evenly. Give the patient two *qián* each dose, once in the morning and once in the evening, swallowed with boiled water. The patient will recover in two days.

又方：麥粉（五錢），炒黃研末，白湯調服，不過一二次，即止。

Another formula: Stir-fry *mài fěn* (five *qián*) until yellow, then grind it into a [finer] powder. Mix with *bái tāng*[66] and give it to the patient. It will stop in not more than one or two doses.

---

66. 白湯 *bái tāng* can mean a plain bland soup, a soup made with white meat only, or possibly plain boiled water. There is also an herbal formula named *bái tāng*, but this passage is unlikely to refer to that formula.

醉後嘔吐視物顛倒不正
Zuì Hòu Ǒu Tǔ Shì Wù Diān Dǎo Bù Zhèng
Vomiting and Seeing Things Upside-Down
or Crooked After Becoming Intoxicated

甜瓜蒂、藜蘆，右各等分，水煎服，令再嘔吐，即愈。

Boil equal portions of *tián guā dì* and *lí lú* in water and give it to the patient to make him vomit. He will recover.

戒煙四物飲 *Jiè Yān Sì Wù Yǐn*
Drink of Four Ingredients for Cessation of Smoking Opium

四物飲：赤沙糖（一斤）、生甘草（一斤）、川貝母（一兩，去心，研細）、老薑（四兩）。

brown sugar		1 *jīn*
shēng gān cǎo		1 *jīn*
chuān bèi mǔ	remove the core, grind into a powder	1 *liǎng*
old ginger (*lǎo jiāng*)		4 *liǎng*

先用鴉片灰（五錢），熬膏，再入前藥同熬，去渣。如一錢癮者，食藥五錢，逐日減少。並以赤沙糖沖水代茶，即斷。如癮極重者，取已煎之汁重煎之，十杯，煎成一杯，再服必效。

First simmer opium ash (*yā piàn huī*,[67] five *qián*) into a paste. Then add the above medicinals, simmer them together, and remove the dregs. If the patient is a one-*qián* addict, he should eat five *qián* of the medicine. Day by day, decrease it. At the same time, drench brown sugar with water as a substitute for tea, and this will break the addiction. If the addiction is extremely heavy, reboil the already-boiled liquid from ten cups down to one cup. Taking it again will certainly be effective.

---

67. This is the residue left in an opium pipe after it has been used. Some morphine remains in it.

81

有人二十余年老癮，照此戒斷，不可輕視 。

There was someone who was addicted for more than twenty years. He broke the addiction using this formula. Do not underestimate this formula.

又方：南瓜藤取汁，調紅糖 、（ 黃糖亦可 ）飲之，神效 。又已戒煙癮之人，平時多食南瓜，免生別病；否則煙雖戒斷，一二年外，仍有後患 。此西洋秘傳也 。

Another formula: Drink the juice from *nán guā téng* mixed with red sugar (yellow sugar can also be used).[68] This has miraculous effects. Also, someone who has already given up opium addiction should eat *nán guā* often in normal times to avoid developing other diseases. Otherwise, he may still have trouble in the future, after one or two years, even though he has broken the opium addiction. This has been secretly transmitted from the West.

又方：粟殼（ 斤半蜜炙透 ）、台黨參（ 一斤 ）、川杜仲（ 六兩 ）、鹽砂仁（ 二兩研末 ）、炮薑（ 五兩 ）、廣陳皮（ 二兩 ）、真雲苓（ 四兩 ）、焦查肉（ 六兩 ）。

Another formula:

sù ké	粟殼	honey-fried until the honey penetrates	1.5 *jīn*
tái dǎng shēn	台黨參		1 *jīn*
chuān dù zhòng	川杜仲		6 *liǎng*
yán shā rén	鹽砂仁	ground into a powder	2 *liǎng*
pào jiāng	炮薑		5 *liǎng*
guǎng chén pí	廣陳皮		2 *liǎng*
Genuine *yún ling*	雲苓		4 *liǎng*
jiāo [shān] zhá ròu	焦[山]查肉		6 *liǎng*

用水一大鍋，煮半日許，將渣瀝淨，再用微火熬成膏，將砂仁末，攪入磁罐收貯 。癮發時，隨癮之大小，白開水化服 。無論癮之新久，無不斷也 。

---

68. *Huáng táng* is literally yellow sugar, but it is what we might call light brown sugar. *Hóng táng* translates literally as red sugar and is equivalent to our brown sugar.

Boil the above [except the *shā rén* powder] in a big cauldron of water for about a half a day. Filter out the dregs. Then use a low fire to simmer the liquid into syrup. Stir in the *shā rén* powder and store it in a porcelain jar. When the addiction manifests, mix the syrup with plain boiled water and have the patient take it. The dose should be based on the size of the addiction. No matter whether the addiction is new or long term, all are able to break it.

若癮來時腹痛，加肉桂（　一兩　）、炙草（　一兩　）。咳嗽，加
苦杏仁（　一兩，研成泥　）、麥冬（　一兩　）、蜂蜜（　四兩　）、
陳皮（　二兩　）。渾身發攤，黨參（　加倍用　）。瀉者，加茯
苓、炮薑（　加倍用　）。腰痛，加杜仲（　三兩　）。不欲食，加
砂仁（　一兩　）。氣下墜者，黨參（　加倍用　）。大便滯者，加
蜂蜜（　三兩　）。肝氣發者，加當歸（　四兩　）、薑香附
（　二兩　）。

- If there is abdominal pain when the addiction comes on, add *ròu guì* (one *liǎng*) and *zhì cǎo* (one *liǎng*).
- For cough, add *kǔ xìng rén* (one *liǎng*, ground into a paste), *mài dōng* (one *liǎng*), honey (four *liǎng*), and *chén pí* (two *liǎng*).
- If the body is paralysed from head to foot, double the amount of *dǎng shēn*.
- For diarrhea, add *fú líng* and double the amount of *pào jiāng*.
- For low back pain, add *dù zhòng* (three *liǎng*).
- If there is no desire to eat, add *shā rén* (one *liǎng*).
- For qì sagging down, double the amount of *dǎng shēn*.
- For stagnation of stool, add honey (three *liǎng*).
- For manifestations of liver qì, add *dāng guī* (four *liǎng*) and *jiāng xiāng fù* (two *liǎng*).

又方：真淮山藥、茯苓、法夏、杜仲、鶴虱、旋覆花
（　絹包　）、款冬花（　各三錢　）、加大煙灰（　三錢　），右以河
水熬成一麭碗，去渣，分十餘次，兌酒服。早癮早服，晚癮
晚服，甚效。

Another formula:

Genuine *huái shān yào*	淮山藥	3 *qián*
fú líng	茯苓	3 *qián*

fǎ xià	法夏		3 *qián*
dù zhòng	杜仲		3 *qián*
hè shī	鶴虱		3 *qián*
xuán fù huā	旋覆花	wrapped in thick silk	3 *qián*
kuǎn dōng huā	款冬花		3 *qián*
yā piàn huī	鴉片灰		3 *qián*

右以河水熬成一麪碗，去渣，分十餘次，兌酒服。早癮早服，晚癮晚服，甚效。

Simmer this in river water down to the amount that would fit in a noodle bowl. Remove the dregs, and divide it into ten or more doses. Add liquor and give it to the patient. If the addiction comes on in the morning, he should take it in the morning. If the addiction comes on in the evening, he should take it in the evening. This is extremely effective.

又方：罌粟殼（八錢）、陳皮（八分）、查灰（一錢）、焦朮（五分）、炮薑（八分）、杜仲（一錢）、甘草（二錢）、炙芪（三錢）、香附（七分）、真台黨（一兩）。

Another formula:

yīng sù ké	罌粟殼	8 *qián*
chén pí	陳皮	8 *fēn*
[*shān*] *zhá huī*	[山]查灰	1 *qián*
jiāo zhú	焦朮	5 *fēn*
pào jiāng	炮薑	8 *fēn*
dù zhòng	杜仲	1 *qián*
gān cǎo	甘草	2 *qián*
zhì qí	炙芪	3 *qián*
xiāng fù	香附	7 *fēn*
Genuine *tái dǎng*	台黨	1 *liǎng*

右藥每日一服，服至月餘，其癮必斷。

The patient should take the above medicine once a day for more than a month. The addiction will certainly be broken.

又方：用甘草一味熬膏，調入煙中吸食。二三日，即漸不欲吸。此方最易，既不費錢，又不傷人。斷後並無煙痢之疾。癮深者，照法治之，一月即斷。

Another formula: Simmer one herb, *gān cǎo*, into a paste. Mix it into the opium and suck it in [inhale it]. In two or three days, the addict will gradually lose the desire to inhale [opium]. This is the easiest formula since it is inexpensive and also does not harm the patient. After breaking the addiction, he will not have the disease of opium dysentery.[69] If the addiction is severe, treat it according to this method; it will break the addiction in a month.

又方：頂上台黨（二兩）、金銀花、旋覆花（絹包）、大生地（各五錢）、麥冬、天冬、炒白芍、真雲苓、木瓜（各一錢）、吳萸、柴胡、沙苑（此味以皮貨店為真，各藥店均係假充[70]）、杜仲（各四錢）。

Another formula:

superior quality *tái dǎng*	台黨		2 *liǎng*
jīn yín huā	金銀花		5 *fēn*
xuán fù huā	旋覆花	wrapped in thick silk	5 *fēn*
dà shēng dì	大生地		5 *fēn*
mài dōng	麥冬		1 *qián*
tiān dōng	天冬		1 *qián*
chǎo bái sháo	炒白芍		1 *qián*
genuine *yún líng*	雲苓		1 *qián*
mù guā	木瓜		1 *qián*
wú yú	吳萸		4 *qián*
chái hú	柴胡		4 *qián*
shā yuàn	沙苑	for this herb, take what is sold in a fur or leather store as genuine, every pharmacy substitutes a fake product.	4 *qián*
dù zhòng	杜仲		4 *qián*

69. Opium use frequently causes severe constipation. Withdrawal from opium can result in diarrhea, vomiting, and other digestive tract symptoms.

70. Apparently this herb is used in processing leather or fur.

加煙灰（ 二錢 ），右同熬 。或加紅糖（ 五錢 ），亦可 。以後
每一料，減煙灰（ 五分 ）至第五料，則不用煙灰 。癮重者，
四五料即斷；輕者三料除根 。有人食煙二十餘年，百藥不
效，照此服之，五料即安然戒斷，並無難過之處 。無論早中
晚癮，總於飯前，熱水沖服 。如一錢癮者，每服二錢 。

Add two *qián* of opium ash (*yā piàn huī*), and simmer the above together.
Brown sugar (five *qián*) can also be added. After this, decrease the opium ash
(by five *fēn*) each batch, until the fifth batch. At that time, don't use opium ash.
If the person is heavily addicted, the addiction will be broken after the fourth
or fifth batch. If it is a light addiction, three batches will cure it once and for
all [literally 'eliminate the roots']. There are people who have eaten opium for
more than twenty years and the hundred medicines were not effective. But
when they took five batches of this formula, they peacefully broke the addiction
without difficulty. No matter whether the addiction is in morning, noon, or
evening, always drench the medicine in hot water and have the patient take it
before meals. If it is a one-*qián* addiction, two *qián* should be taken each time.[71]

---

71. This paragraph is found in《 急救易知 》*Jí Jiù Yì Zhī* (Easily Understood
Emergency Treatment) but not in《 驗方新編 》*Yàn Fāng Xīn Biān* (New
Compilation of Proven Formulas).

Chapter 5

人畜蛇蟲咬傷 *Rén Chù Shé Chóng Yǎo Shāng*
Human, Animal, Snake, or Insect Bites

Translator's Note: This chapter is abridged from Volume 13 of《驗方新編》*Yàn Fāng Xīn Biān*.

凡各物咬傷，日久不愈者，人咬傷第二方甘草治之，極效。

Whenever someone has been bitten by something and it doesn't recover in the course of time, the *gān cǎo* formula, which is second under Human Bite Wounds, is extremely effective.

人咬傷 *Rén Yǎo Shāng*
Human Bite Wounds

凡被人咬傷，其牙最毒。若有牙垢入肉，則痛不可忍。咬手指者，指與手掌，俱漸爛落。年久難愈，重者喪命。

Whenever there are wounds from human bites, the teeth are the most toxic. When tartar[72] goes into the flesh, the pain is unendurable. If a finger was bitten, then the fingers, hand and palm all gradually putrefy and drop off. It is difficult to recover, even after years. In serious cases, the victim may lose his life.

無論日久初起，雖至腫爛，總宜用童便（用淘米水洗亦可），洗淨污血。

---

72. Literally, tooth dirt (牙垢 *yá gòu*).

No matter how many days ago it began, even when it has become swollen and putrefied, the foul blood should always be washed away with child's urine (water that has been used to wash rice can also be used).

又方：照前洗淨之後，用甘草自己嚼融濃敷，乾則隨換，日夜不斷，三日必愈，屢試奇驗。並治各物咬傷亦效。

Another formula: After washing it according to the above directions, the patient himself should chew *gān cǎo* until it is soft and apply a thick layer of it on the site. Change it when the *gān cǎo* is dry and do not stop, day and night. In three days the patient will recover. Together, [the washing and the application of *gān cǎo*] are effective for treating various kinds of bites.

有人被鼠咬指，數年不愈，照此洗淨敷治，三日收功，真神方也。

Someone was bitten on the finger by a rat and did not recover for several years. He was treated according to this washing and application method. He achieved success in three days. This is really a miraculous formula.

又方：鱉甲燒灰敷之，奇效。

Another formula: Apply *biē jiǎ* that has been reduced to ashes. This is extraordinarily effective.

又方：先用童便洗淨，用荔枝核焙，研篩細，摻之。外用荔肉蓋貼。雖入水不爛，神效之極。

Another formula: First wash the site with child's urine, then grind and sift stone-baked *lì zhī hé* to make a fine powder and sprinkle it on. Externally cover the site by sticking on *lì ròu*; even if it gets wet, the wound will not putrefy. This has extremely miraculous effects.

虎傷 *Hǔ Shāng*
Tiger Wounds

凡被虎咬傷，血必大出，傷口立時潰爛，疼不可當。急用豬
肉貼之，隨貼隨化，隨化隨換。速用地榆一斤為細末，加入
三七末三兩、苦參末四兩，和勻摻之，隨濕隨摻，血即止而
痛即定。蓋地榆涼血，苦參止痛，三七末止血，合三者之
長，故奏效如神。

Tiger bites bleed a lot, the wound immediately festers, and the pain is unbearable. Quickly stick a piece of pork on the site, and as soon as it is applied, the pork will transform;[73] as soon as it transforms, change it. Quickly use a *jīn* of finely powdered *dì yú*. Add in three *liǎng* of powdered *sān qī* and four *liǎng* of powdered *kǔ shēn*. Blend evenly and sprinkle it on. Sprinkle more on as soon as it becomes moist. The bleeding will then stop and the pain will settle. *Dì yú* cools the blood, *kǔ shēn* stops pain and *sān qī* powder stops bleeding; these are the strong points of the three when combined. Thus it is miraculously effective.

又方：內服生薑汁。外以薑汁洗過，用白礬末敷之。

Another formula: The patient should take *shēng jiāng* juice internally. Externally, apply powdered *bái fán* to it after washing the site with ginger juice.

野狼傷 *Yě Láng Shāng*
Wolf Wounds

乾薑末敷，或胡椒末敷。初覺腫痛，少刻即腫消痛止，三日
而安。

Apply powdered *gān jiāng* or *hú jiāo* to it. Initially the patient will feel swelling and pain, but in a short while, the swelling disperses and the pain stops. He will be secure in three days.

---

73. It seems the pork changes color or texture when it is applied to the wound.

癲犬咬傷 *Diān Quǎn Yǎo Shāng*
Mad Dog Bites

此症最險，七日一發。發時天本無風，病者俱覺風大，入帳蒙頭躲避，此非吉兆。過三七之日，無此畏風情形，方為可治。

This disease is most dangerous! It manifests in seven days [from the time of the bite]. At the time it manifests, there is no wind in heaven itself [but these] patients all strongly feel wind. They go into an enclosed place, cover their heads, and hide; this is not an auspicious sign. But it can be treated if three times seven [twenty-one] days pass without this state of fearing of wind.

被咬時，先看頭頂，如有紅髮二、三根，趕緊拔去，最為緊要。

At the time the patient was bitten, the first sign is that two or three red hairs appear at the vertex of the head. Quickly pull them out. This is most crucial.

隨於無風處，以冷茶洗淨污血。用杏仁搗融敷之。內服韭菜汁一碗，隔七日再服一碗，四十九日，共服七碗。

Then in a place where there is no wind, wash away the foul blood from the wound with cold tea. Pound *xìng rén* until soft and apply it to the bite. Internally the patient should take a bowl of *jiǔ cài* juice. Every seven days, he should take another bowl of it. At forty-nine days, he should have consumed seven bowls altogether.

傷口上再用煮熟雞蛋白蓋上，用艾絨在上燒數十次。

Also cover the wound with boiled chicken egg whites. Burn moxa floss on top several tens of times.

百日內忌鹽醋；一年內忌豬肉、魚腥、酒色；終身忌食狗肉、蠶豆、紅飯豆；方得保全；否則十有九死。

The patient should avoid salt and vinegar for the next hundred days, and he should avoid pork, fish, and sensual pursuits [liquor and women] for the next year. Further, he should avoid eating dog meat, broad beans (*cán dòu*), and red rice beans (*hóng fàn dòu*)[74] for the rest of his life. This will give complete protection. Without doing this, nine out of ten will die.

又方：地骨皮（ 即枸杞根 ），搗爛，熬酒服，一二日當茶飲，永無後患 。

Another formula: *dì gǔ pí* (meaning the root of *gǒu qǐ*) pounded to a pulp. Simmer it in liquor and have the patient take it. The patient should drink tea[75] constantly for one or two days and there will never be future suffering.

家犬咬傷 *Jiā Quǎn Yǎo Shāng*
Family Dog Bites

胡椒（ 研細末 ）敷之，雖傷重，亦不過數日，收功，惟初敷必痛而且腫；少刻，痛止腫消 。

Grind *hú jiāo* into a fine powder and apply it. Even if the wound is severe it will successfully contract[76] in not more than a few days. It will only hurt and swell up when the powder is initially applied; a moment later, the pain will stop and the swelling will disperse.

有人被犬咬傷，血流不止，用此藥隨敷隨流，敷至第三次後血止，數日而愈，其效如神 。

Someone was bitten by a dog and could not stop bleeding. The bleeding stopped after he applied this medicine for the third time and he recovered in several days. Its effects are like a miracle.

又方：用木一截，向傷處指定，在木尾燒之，問其痛否？不痛乃愈 。犬本屬土，此木能克土之意也 。

---

74. 紅飯豆 *hóng fàn dòu* are also called 赤小豆 *chì xiǎo dòu*.
75. Theae Folium.
76. Close up.

Another formula: Point a length of wood toward the affected site. Burn the tail end of the wood and ask the patient whether or not it still hurts. He will recover if it does not hurt. The idea is that dog corresponds to earth and this wood is able to control earth.

又方：甜杏仁去皮尖，嚼爛敷之 。

Another formula: Remove the skin and tips from *tián xìng rén*, chew it into a pulp, and apply it.

馬咬傷 *Mǎ Yǎo Shāng*
Horse Bites

白煮豬肉一大片，同飯 。本人自嚼，貼患處，立時止痛，即 愈 。

One big slice of pork boiled in plain[77] water together with rice. I myself was bitten and stuck pork that was cooked this way on the affected site. The pain stopped immediately and the wound promptly recovered.[78]

又方：益母草搗爛，調醋烘熱，敷之 。

Another formula: Pound *yì mǔ cǎo* to a pulp. Mix it with vinegar, heat it up, and apply it.

豬咬傷 *Zhū Yǎo Shāng*
Pig Bites

上龜板炙研細，麻油調搽，即愈 。

Process superior quality *guī bǎn*. Finely powder and mix it with sesame oil. The patient will recover after rubbing it in.

---

77. Unsalted, unspiced.

78. This story describes the experience of the author, Bào Xiāng'áo.

又方：熟松香，貼傷處，數日愈。

Another formula: Stick processed *sōng xiāng* onto the wound. It will recover in a few days.

猿猴抓傷 *Yuán Hóu Zhuā Shāng*
Mauling by Apes or Monkeys

金毛狗脊焙研末，摻之。或用麻油調搽，立愈。

Stone-bake and powder *jīn máo gǒu jí* and sprinkle it on. Or mix it with sesame oil and rub it in. The patient will immediately recover.

貓咬傷 *Māo Yǎo Shāng*
Cat Bites

用薄荷煎水洗之。或用川椒煎水洗之。

Boil *bò hé* in water and wash the site. Or boil *chuān jiāo* in water and wash it.

鼠咬傷 *Shǔ Yǎo Shāng*
Rat or Mouse Bites

荔枝嚼融敷，即愈。或用貓兒口水搽之。

The patient will recover after chewing *lì zhī* until it is soft and applying it. Or rub the saliva of kittens into it.

蛇咬傷 *Shé Yǎo Shāng*
Snake Bites

煙精膏 *Yān Jīng Gāo* (Smoke Essence Paste)

凡遇毒蛇咬傷，惡毒攻心，半日必死。急取煙筒內煙油，用
冷水洗出，飲一二碗，受毒重者，其味必甜而不辣，以多飲
為佳。傷口痛甚者，用煙油搽擦，必出。此為蛇咬第一仙
方，切不可疑而自誤。

Whenever a poisonous snake bite occurs, malign toxins attack the heart, and
the victim will die within half a day. Quickly wash out tar from the inside a
chimney with cold water, and have the patient drink one or two bowls of it. If
the victim received a serious dose of venom, it will taste sweet and not spicy.
Drinking a lot of it is good. If the pain at the wound is severe, rub the tar into it.
[The venom] will come out. This is the best prescription of the immortals for
snake bite; be sure not to doubt it or you will damage your own interests.

道光八九年間，粵西崇善縣地方，有農人被毒蛇咬住，繞纏
不放，急服煙油水數碗，並以煙油滴蛇口內，蛇即松口落地
而死，其人無恙。

A farmer was bitten by a poisonous snake in 1828 or 1829 (Emperor
Dàoguāng's eight or nineth year), in Yuèxi (Western Guǎngdōng province),
Chóngshàn county. The snake wound around him and would not let go. He
quickly drank several bowls of chimney tar water and simultaneously dripped
chimney tar into the snake's mouth. The snake then let go, fell to the ground,
and died, and the person was safe and sound.

又方：有人被蛇咬傷，即刻昏死，臂脹如臌少頃，遍身皮脹
黃黑色。一道人以新汲水調香白芷末一斤，灌之，覺臍中聲
響，黃同水從傷口流出，良久便愈。

Another formula: Someone was bitten by a snake and immediately fell into a
coma. In a short while, his arm swelled up like a drum and the skin of his entire
body became swollen and turned yellow and black. A Dàoist mixed newly-
drawn water with one *jīn* of *xiāng bái zhī* and poured it into the victim. Sounds

were heard in his umbilicus and yellowish water flowed out from the wound. He recovered after a long while.

又方：川貝母末，酒調，盡量飲之，少刻，酒自傷口流出，候流盡，以渣敷上，垂死，亦效。

Another formula: Powdered *chuān bèi mǔ* mixed with liquor. The patient should drink as much as possible. A moment later, liquor will flow out from the wound. Wait until the flow has finished, and apply the dregs to the site. It is even effective for those who are near death.

又方：用兩刀在水內相磨，取水飲之，雖痛苦欲死可救。

Another formula: Grind two knives against each other in water, and have the victim drink this water. He can be rescued even if he is suffering a lot and is about to die.

又方：用雞蛋破一孔，對傷口按住，少刻，蛋內色即變黑，黑則又換，以蛋色不變為止（要雞蛋，不要鴨蛋）。

Another formula: Break a hole in a chicken's egg and press it over the wound. In a little while, the color inside the egg will turn black. Keep changing the egg when it turns black until it no longer changes (it is important to use a chicken egg, not a duck egg).

又方：五靈脂（一錢）、雄黃（五錢）。右共為細末，每服二錢，酒調服；不飲酒者，開水調服。並敷傷處，雖至垂危，亦可救也。

Another formula: Finely powder *wǔ líng zhī* (one *qián*) and *xióng huáng* (five *qián*) together. The patient should take two *qián* mixed with liquor each dose. If the patient does not drink liquor, mix it with boiled water for him to take. At the same time, apply it to the wound. Even if the patient has reached a critical stage, this can still rescue him.

又方：嫩黃荊葉（采取生者以七葉為佳）搗汁敷之，極效。

Another formula: Crush tender *huáng jīng yè* (it is good to pick it fresh and use seven leaves) to extract the juice and apply it. This is extremely effective.

蜈蚣咬傷 *Wú Gōng Yǎo Shāng*
Centipede Bites

指甲，磨水敷，立效如神，萬無一失。

Grind finger nails in water and apply it. This is immediately effective like a miracle and not one in ten-thousand will be lost.

有人被蜈蚣咬傷，其色碧綠，腫大如碗，痛不可忍，百藥隨敷隨乾，其毒不散，後用此方治之，應手而愈。此法最為簡便，毋庸第二方也。各項毒物咬傷，雖未試過，想亦可治。

When someone was bitten by a centipede, his complexion became dark green, he swelled up like a bowl, and the pain was unendurable. He applied a hundred different medicines in vain, but the toxins did not disperse. After treating it with this formula, his recovery went smoothly. This method is the most simple and convenient; there is no need for a second formula. Although I have not yet tried it for each and every type of toxic bite, I feel it can treat them all.

蠍螫傷 *Xiē Zhē Shāng*
Scorpion Stings

雄者傷人，痛在一處；雌者傷人，痛牽遍體。用井底泥敷之，乾則再換，或用新汲水，以青布隨痛處搭之，乾則再換，亦效。

When male scorpions sting people, the pain is in the one site. When the female stings people, the pain is drawn into the whole body. Apply mud from the bottom of a well to the sting, and change it when it becomes dry. Drape black cloth moisted with newly-drawn water over the painful site. Change it when the cloth gets dry. This is also effective.

又方：用二味拔毒散，更妙。

Another formula: Use *Èr Wèi Bá Dú Sàn* (Two Ingredient Powder to Pull Out Toxins).[79] This is even more wonderful.

又方：用木碗蓋於痛處，過半日即愈，神驗之至。

Cover the painful site with a wooden bowl; recovery will come after half a day. This gives extremely miraculous experiences.

壁虎咬傷 *Bì Hǔ Yǎo Shāng*
Gecko (or House Lizard) Bites

桑葉煎濃汁，調白礬末敷之。或照前蜈蚣咬傷方治之。

Boil *sāng yè* into a concentrated liquid. Mix it with powdered *bái fán* and apply it. Or treat it according to the above formula for centipede bites.

黃蜂傷 *Huáng Fēng Shāng*
Wasp Stings

蚯蚓糞，井水調敷，其痛立止。

Mix earthworm excrement[80] with well water and apply it. The pain will stop immediately.

又方：芋頭梗搗融敷，極效。

Another formula: Pound *yù tóu* (taro) stalks until soft and apply it. This is extremely effective.

---

79. 二味拔毒散 *Èr Wèi Bá Dú Sàn* (Two Ingredient Powder to Pull Out Toxins): This formula is given in Volume 11: 治一切毒蟲咬傷，無論腫痛瘙癢，敷之立止，其效神速。雄黃、枯礬，各等分為末，先用薑汁洗淨，用茶調敷。 It treats all types of toxic *chóng* bites. Whether there is swelling, pain, or itching, it will immediately stop when this formula is applied. Its effects are miraculously quick. Mix equal portions of powdered *xióng huáng* and *kū fán*. First clean the site with ginger juice, mix the powder with tea and apply it.
80. 蚯蚓糞 *qiū yǐn fèn* (earthworm excrement) probably means worm castings.

又方：用二味拔毒散，敷之，最效 。

Another formula: Apply *Èr Wèi Bá Dú Sàn* (Two Ingredient Powder to Pull Out Toxins) to it. This is most effective.

射工溪毒傷 *Shè Gōng Xī Dú Shāng*
Shè Gōng (Archer) and Stream Toxins

此水中射工也，又有樹上毛蟲，亦名射工者，見後毛蟲傷
方。射工一名溪鬼蟲，又名射影，又名水弩。出南方有溪毒
處 。

This is the aquatic *shè gōng*; there is also a caterpillar on trees that is named *shè gōng*, described in the next item under Caterpillar Damage. Other names for *shè gōng* are *xī guǐ chóng* (Stream Ghost Bug), *shè yǐng* (Shoot Shadows), or *shuǐ nǔ* (Water Crossbow). It comes from the south, where there are places with stream toxins.

長二三寸，寬寸許，形扁，前寬後窄，腹頓背硬，如蟬又如
鼈。六七月甲下有翅，能飛作鉍鉍聲。寬頭尖嘴，嘴頭有角
如爪，長一二分，有六足，如蟹足，兩足在嘴下，大而一
爪，四足在腹下，小而雙爪。口有弩形，以氣射人影，去人
三、四步即中。令人發瘡，不治即死 。

The *shè gōng* is two or three *cùn* long and about a *cùn* wide. Its body is flat with a broad front but a narrow back. The abdomen is soft but the back is hard. It looks like a cicada, and also like a soft-shelled turtle. During the sixth or seventh lunar month, it has wings beneath its shell. It is able to fly and makes a "*bì bì*" sound. Its head is broad with a pointed beak. The end of the beak has a claw-like horn one or two *fēn* long. It has six crab-like legs. Two legs are under its beak, big with one claw. Four legs are under its abdomen, small with twin claws. The mouth is in the form of a crossbow. It shoots qì at human shadows. When the person walks three or four steps, he is hit. It makes sores erupt on people. If these are not treated, they will die.

病有四種，初得皆如傷寒，或似中惡。一種遍身有黑靨子，四邊微紅，犯之如刺；一種作瘡，久則穿陷；一種突起如石；一種如火燒狀。

There are four types of this disease. Initially all resemble cold damage. Sometimes it seems like malignity stroke. In one type, the entire body has black spots that are slightly red on the edges. They feel like thorns to the person who suffers it. One type makes sores that penetrate and cave in after a long time. One type suddenly rises up like stones. One type resembles the shape of burning flames.

又有溪毒中人，一名中水，一名中溪，一名水病。似射工而不見形。春月多有此病症，頭痛惡寒，狀如傷寒，二三日，腹中生蟲，食人下部，漸食五臟，注下不禁，雖良醫難治。

People can also be struck by stream toxins, which are also called water strike, stream strike, or water disease. This is similar to *shè gōng*, but invisible. During spring months, there are many cases of this disease. It seems like cold damage, with headache and aversion to cold. In two or three days, worms grow in the abdomen and consume the person's lower [private] parts. It gradually consumes the five viscera, with downpour diarrhea and incontinence of stool. This is difficult to treat, even for a good doctor.

初得則下部有瘡紅赤，形如截肉，為陽毒，最急；若瘡如蟲嚙為陰毒，其勢稍緩，皆能殺人，過二十日不治，方家用藥。與傷寒、瘟病相似。須用蒼耳草絞汁，服一二升；並用棉蘸汁，濃敷下部。或以小蒜煮微熱湯（不可大熱，大熱則無力）洗之。若身發赤斑，其毒已出也。

In the initial stages, the lower [private] parts develop sores and redness. Yáng toxins look like chopped meat; this is most urgent. Yīn toxin sores look like insects have been gnawing; this condition is somewhat slower. Either one can kill people if a skilled doctor does not treat it with herbal medicine within twenty days. It resembles cold damage or warm disease.[81] You must wring out the juice from *cāng ěr cǎo* and have the patient take one or two *shēng*. At the same time, dip cotton in the juice and apply a thick layer on the lower parts. Some boil

---

81. Here, the text says 瘟病 *wēn bìng* (scourge disease). This is probably a typographical error for 溫病 *wēn bìng* (warm disease).

99

xiǎo suàn and wash the region with the slightly hot decoction (it cannot be too hot or it will lack strength). If the body erupts in red macules, the toxins have already left.

又方：用鹽梅裹含之，亦可 。

Another formula: You can also hold a salted plum inside the mouth.

又方：知母連根葉研末服；或投水絞汁飲一二升；煮湯洗浴，亦佳 。

Another formula: Grind *zhī mǔ*, including the roots and leaves, into a powder and have the patient take it. Some throw it in water, wring out the juice and drink one or two *shēng*. It is also good to boil it into a decoction and bathe in it.

又方：蒼耳草嫩苗，取汁，和酒溫灌之，其渣厚敷傷處，甚效 。

Another formula: Blend the juice from delicate seedlings of *cāng ěr cǎo* with liquor. Warm it and pour it in. Apply a thick layer of the dregs to the damaged site. This is extremely effective.

又方：芥菜子末，和酒厚敷，半日止痛 。

Another formula: Powder mustard seeds (*jiè cài zǐ*). Blend them with liquor and apply a thick layer. The pain will stop in half a day.

又方：馬齒莧搗汁一升服，以渣敷之，日四 、五次 。

Another formula: Crush *mǎ chǐ xiàn* to extract the juice and have the patient take one *shēng*. Apply the dregs to the site four or five times a day.

毛蟲傷 *Máo Chóng Shāng*
Caterpillar Damage

毛蟲，俗名楊辣子，又名射工，能放毛射人 。初癢次痛，勢如火燒，久則外癢內痛，骨肉皆爛，諸藥罔效 。用豆豉搗融，清油調敷，少時，則有毛出 。去豆豉，用白芷煎湯洗之。如肉已爛，用海螵蛸末摻之，即愈。

The common name of this caterpillar is *yáng là zǐ* (Cayenne Pepper from the Poplar). It is also called *shè gōng* (Archer) because it is able to shoot hairs into people. It initially itches, but then becomes painful and feels like burning fire. After a long time, there is external itching and internal pain. The bones and flesh both putrefy. No medicine is effective. Pound *dòu chǐ* until soft, mix it with clear oil[82] and apply it. In a little while, the hairs will come out. Remove the *dòu chǐ*. Boil *bái zhǐ* into a decoction and wash it. If the flesh has already putrefied, it will recover after sprinkling on powdered *hǎi piāo xiāo*.

又方：二味拔毒散，最效。

Another formula: *Èr Wèi Bá Dú Sàn* (Two Ingredient Powder to Pull Out Toxins) is most effective.

又方：先以水洗之，隨用馬齒莧搗爛敷之，一二次即愈。或以熟蜜搽之，亦效。

Another formula: First wash it with water, then pound *mǎ chǐ xiàn* into a pulp, and apply it. It will recover after one or two applications. Or it is also effective to rub cooked honey into it.

蜘蛛傷 Zhī Zhū Shāng
Spider (Aranea) Bites

有人蜘蛛咬傷，腹大如臌，遍身生絲，飲白羊乳數日而愈。

The abdomen of some people who are bitten by spiders become swollen like a drum and the entire body grows [visible] veins. They will recover when they drink the milk of white goats for several days.

又方：飲好酒至醉，則肉中自出小蟲而愈。

---

82. Wiseman says 清油 *qīng yóu* (clear oil) refers to soy sauce. According to other dictionaries, it refers to vegetable oil, tea oil or simply clear oil without sediments.

Another formula: When the patient drinks good liquor until intoxicated, a small *chóng* will crawl out from the flesh and he will recover.

又方：熱甜酒洗之即消 。

Another formula: It will disperse when you wash it in sweet liquor (*tián jiǔ*) that has been heated.

蟢蛛傷 *Xǐ Zhū Shāng*
Spider (Uroctea compactilis or Uroctea lesserti) Bites

此物形以蜘蛛而大，一名壁錢，又名壁鏡，又名蟢子 。時作白窠如錢大貼壁上，咬人最毒，不治必死。用桑樹枝燒枯，煎濃汁，調白礬末敷之，極效 。

This thing is shaped like a spider (*zhī zhū*) but larger. It is also called *bì qián*, *bì jìng*, or *xǐ zǐ*. Sometimes it makes white burrows the size of a coin in a wall or cliff. Its bites are very toxic for people, and if not treated, the person will die. Roast mulberry branches (*sāng shù zhī*) until they are dried out, and boil them into a concentrated liquid. Mix with powdered *bái fán* and apply it. This is extremely effective.

多足蟲傷 *Duō Zú Chóng Shāng*
Many-Legged Insect Bites

一名蠼螋 。以尿射人，誤中其毒，令人皮膚起燎漿泡，痛如火烙。初如飯粒 。次如豆大 。若不早治，傷處周圍交合，則難救 。急用棉蘸熱鹽水敷，數次，即消 。甚者則毒延及遍身，瘙癢不止，宜用二味拔毒散敷之，神效 。或用大黃，末數亦效 。

Also named *qú sōu*.[83] It shoots people with its urine. Burning blisters rise up on a person's skin when he is accidentally struck by its toxins. The pain is like a

---

83. 多足蟲 *duō zú chóng* should refer to millipede, but 蠼螋 *qú sōu* means earwig. Therefore, it is unclear which type of insect bite this section treats.

fiery brand. Initially [the blisters] are the size of grains of rice, and then they become the size of beans. Once the surrounding injured sites grow and meet each other, it is difficult to save the person without early treatment. It will disperse if you quickly dip cotton in hot salt water and apply it several times. In serious cases, the toxins involve the whole body and there is incessant itching. *Èr Wèi Bá Dú Sàn* should be applied to it, as this has miraculous effects. Some apply powdered *dà huáng* to it several times, which is also effective.

蚯蚓毒 *Qiū Yǐn Dú*
Earthworm (Pheretima) Toxins

又名地龍。凡受蚯蚓毒，形如麻瘋，髮眉脫落，或夜間身體作鳴。急以鹽湯，或石灰煎湯，時時洗之，其毒自去。

This is also called *dì lóng*. Whenever someone has received earthworm toxins, it appears like numbing wind.[84] His hair and eyebrows fall off, and sometimes at night, his body makes sounds. Quickly boil salt or lime (*shí huī*) in water and frequently wash him with it. The toxins will automatically be removed.

蠶咬傷 *Cán Yǎo Shāng*
Silkworm Bites

凡蠶嚙人，毒入肉中，令人發寒熱。以家用苧麻葉搗汁塗之，神效。

Whenever silkworms gnaw on people, their toxins enter the flesh, making people present with [aversion to] cold and heat. Crush household rush leaves (*zhù má yè*) to extract the juice and smear it on. This has miraculous effects.

又方：蜜調麝香敷之，亦效。

Another formula: Apply honey mixed with *shè xiāng* to it. This is also effective.

---

84. 麻瘋 *má fēng* (leprosy).

狐尿刺毒 *Hú Niào Cì Dú*
Fox Urine Thorn Toxins[85]

一名狐狸刺。由螳螂盛暑交媾，精汁染於諸物，乾久有毒，
人之手足誤觸之，則成此患。初起紅紫斑點，肌膚乾燥，悶
腫，焮痛，不眠，至十日後腐開，則瘡口日寬。

Another name is *hú lí cì* (Fox Thorns). This condition is due to the mating of
the mantis (*táng láng*) in midsummer. The juice of its essence stains everything, and it becomes toxic after being dried for a long time. This condition
develops when someone's hands or feet accidentally touch it. Initially red-
purple spots arise, the flesh and skin dry out, then there is oppression, swelling,
burning pain, and insomnia. When ten days have passed, putrefaction begins;
the sores open up and get wider by the day.

初起未潰者，以蒲公英連根煎濃，溫洗，若得鮮者，搗汁塗
之，更妙。內服黃連解毒湯，即愈。若已潰爛，照前甘草諸
方治之，或照癰毒諸方治之。

Initially, before it has festered, boil *pú gōng yīng*, including the roots until it is
concentrated, and use this as a warm wash. If you can get fresh *pú gōng yīng*,
crush it to extract the juice and smear it on. This is even more wonderful. The
patient will recover after taking *Huáng Lián Jiě Dú Tāng*[86] internally. If it has
already festered, treat it according to the various *gān cǎo* formulas mentioned
above [see the section on Human Bite Wounds]. Or treat it according to the
various formulas for abscesses and toxins.

---

85. One explanation for this name is that a fox may urinate on a plant with
thorns. If someone is then pricked by the thorn, he will develop swelling,
inflammation, and pain in the joints of the hands or feet, depending on whether
he touched it or stepped on it. However, here it is a condition with similar
symptoms caused by an insect.

86. 黃連解毒湯 *Huáng Lián Jiě Dú Tāng*: This formula was first described
in《肘後備急方》*Zhǒu Hòu Bèi Jí Fāng* (Emergency Formulas to Keep up
your Sleeve) by 葛洪 Gé Hóng (281-341), but it received its name in《外台
秘要》*Wài Tái Mì Yào* (Essential Secrets from a Border Official) written in
752 by 王濤 Wáng Tāo. See formula in appendix on p. 200.

各項毒蟲咬傷 *Gè Xiàng Dú Chóng Yǎo Shāng*
Various Toxic Chóng Bites[87]

用二味拔毒散敷之，其效甚速。

Apply *Èr Wèi Bá Dú Sàn*. It is extremely effective and fast.

又方：照前甘草方敷之，神效。

Another formula: Apply the *gān cǎo* formula mentioned above. This has miraculous effects.

---

87. 蟲 *chóng*: A reminder here that *chóng* can mean various types of creep-crawly things, not just bugs and worms.

Chapter 6

湯火傷 *Tāng Huǒ Shāng*
Scalds and Burns

Translator's Note: This chapter is abridged from Volume 13 of 《 驗方 新編 》 *Yàn Fāng Xīn Biān*, except the taro formula at the end of this chapter which came from *Jí Jiù Yì Zhī* 《 急救易知 》 (Easily Understood Emergency Treatment).

湯泡火傷 *Tāng Pào Huǒ Shāng*
Scalds, Blisters, and Burns

凡湯泡、火傷，無論輕重，急用童便灌之，以免火毒攻心。或用白沙糖熱水調服。或用蜂蜜調熱水灌之，均可。

No matter how serious, whenever there are scalds, blisters, or burns, quickly pour child's urine into the patient to prevent fire toxins from attacking the heart; or have him drink white granulated sugar mixed with hot water. You can also mix honey with hot water and pour it into the patient.

第一不可用冷水及井泥溝泥等物。即使痛極難受，亦必忍耐。倘誤用冷水淋之，則熱氣內逼。輕則爛入筋骨，手足彎縮，纏綿難愈；重則直攻入心，必難救矣。

Number one: You cannot use things such as cold water, or mud from a well or ditch. Even if the pain is extreme and difficult to bear, you must still show restraint; if you mistakenly pour cold water on the site, the hot qì will be forced inside. If this is a light case, putrefaction will develop in the sinews and bones,

106

the hands and feet will bend and contract, and it will linger and become difficult to cure. When it is severe, the hot qì directly attacks the heart and it is difficult to save the patient.

先用真麻油敷之，再用糯米淘水，去米取汁，加真麻油一茶鍾，多加更妙，用箸子順攪一二千下，可以挑起成絲，用舊筆蘸油搭上，立刻止痛。愈後並無疤痕，神效無比。

First apply genuine sesame oil to the site. Then wash glutinous rice and strain it, reserving the water. Add a tea cup of genuine sesame oil. Adding more sesame oil is even more wonderful. Stir it clockwise with chopsticks one or two thousand times until it can make threads when you raise up the chopsticks. Dip an old brush in the oil and apply it to the burn. It will immediately stop the pain. After recovery, there will not be a scar. This has incomparable miraculous effects.

又方：先用真桐油（真麻油亦可）敷之。敷後上加食鹽少許，再用生大黃研末摻上，立刻清涼止痛。愈後亦無疤痕。

Another formula: First apply genuine *tóng yóu* to the site (genuine sesame oil can also be used.). After applying it, add a little table salt on top, then sprinkle powdered raw *dà huáng* on top. This will immediately clear, cool, and stop pain, and there will not be a scar after recovery.

又方：清涼膏：新出窖石灰，用冷水化開（水宜多，不宜少）次日水面上，結一層如薄冰樣者，取起，以真桐油和入，調極濃厚，敷之，立刻清涼止痛，日敷三五次。無論初起日久，皆效。

Another formula: *Qīng Liáng Gāo* (Clearing Cooling Paste): Dilute newly-emitted lime (*shí huī*) from the cellar with cold water (you should use a lot of water, not a little). The next day a layer that appears like thin ice will develop on the surface of the water. Pick it up, and blend it into genuine *tóng yóu* until it is extremely concentrated and thick. Apply it to immediately clear, cool, and stop the pain. Apply it three or five times a day. This is effective for everything, no matter how it began.

又方：先用麻油熬滾，次入白蠟熬數滾，再入白蜜熬勻，放水中半日，拔去火氣，用鴨毛調敷，其痛即止。若傷重者並可內服，不至攻心。

Another formula: First bring sesame oil to a rolling simmer. Next add white wax and simmer for several rollings. Then add white honey until it simmers uniformly. Place [the pot] in water for half a day to draw out the fire qì [to let it cool]. The pain will stop when you apply it with a duck feather. If the damage is serious, this can also be taken internally at the same time,[88] so [the fire qì] does not reach the state of attacking the heart.

又方：用蚶子殼（ 又名瓦楞子 ），煅枯，研極細末，配冰片少許。濕則摻敷；乾處麻油調搽數次。

Another formula: Calcine *hān zǐ ké* until it is dried up, then grind it into an extremely fine powder. Mix in a little *bīng piàn*. If the affected site is moist, sprinkle it on, or mix it with sesame oil and rub it onto a dry site several times.

又方：湯火傷治不得法，以致焮赤腫痛，毒腐成膿，用麻油（ 四兩 ）、當歸（ 一兩入麻油內煎焦去渣 ），再入黃蠟（ 一兩 ）攪化，隔水拔火氣，以布攤貼，立能止痛生肌，神效之至。

Another formula: Method for untreated scalds and burns that have become scorching, red, swollen, and painful, with toxins putrifying into pus. Use sesame oil (four *liǎng*) and *dāng guī* (one *liǎng*, add it into the sesame oil, boil until burnt, and remove the dregs). Then add beeswax (one *liǎng*), stirring until it melts. Place [the pot] in water to draw out the fire qì [to let it cool]. Spread it on cloth and stick it on. It is able to immediately stop pain and engender flesh and has extremely miraculous effects.

又方：人乳和鹽敷之。

Another formula: Apply human milk blended with salt.

以上各方，簡便神效，雖傷及遍身，勢在垂危，或潰爛已久，均有奇效。

---

88. Perhaps omitting the wax.

The above formulas are simple, convenient, and miraculously effective. Even if the damage covers the entire body and it is a critical case, perhaps already festering for a long time, all these formulas have extraordinary effects.

又方：蟲蛀竹灰，平時收存，用時，以麻油調搽，極效。

Another formula: In normal times, save the dust that comes out of bamboo which has been damaged by insects. At the time of use, mix it with sesame oil and rub it in. This is extremely effective.

又方：茶葉嚼爛，敷之，立愈。

Another formula: Chew tea leaves until soft and apply them. It will immediately recover.

又方：真麻油（二斤）、生大黃（半斤切片）。銅鍋熬至藥色焦黑，瓦罐連渣收貯，遇湯火傷，用雞毛蘸油搽之。止痛如神，二日即愈。平時預製，可備急用。

Another formula: Genuine sesame oil (two *jīn*) and *shēng dà huáng* (a half *jīn*, sliced). Simmer it in a copper pot until the herbs become burnt black, and store it in an earthen jar, including the dregs. If you encounter a scald or burn, dip a chicken feather in the oil and apply it to the skin. It stops pain like a miracle! The patient will recover in two days. Make it before you need it so you are prepared for emergencies.

火爆傷眼 *Huǒ Bào Shāng Yǎn*
Injury to the Eyes due to a Fiery Explosion

三七葉搗汁點入數次，即愈。或用三七磨水滴入，亦可，屢試如神。又跌打損傷打傷眼睛，南瓜方亦效。

Crush *sān qī* leaves to extract the juice. The patient will recover after dripping it into the eyes several times. *Sān qī* can also be ground in water and dripped in. This has been tried repeatedly and works like a miracle! The pumpkin formula given under Damage to the Eyes from a Beating in the [next] chapter on Traumatic Injury is also effective.

湯火傷立刻止痛方 *Tāng Huǒ Shāng Lì Kè Zhǐ Tòng Fāng*
Formula to Immediately Stop Pain from Scalds and Burns

生芋艿搗融，敷傷處，芋熱再換，數次即愈，立能止痛拔
毒，雖極重，亦不至潰爛。

Pound fresh taro until soft and apply it to the damaged site. When the taro becomes hot, change it. After several times, the patient will recover. It can immediately stop the pain and pull out the toxins, even if the case is extremely serious. Nor will it develop ulceration.

Chapter 7

跌打損傷 *Siē Dǎ Sǔn Shāng*
Traumatic Injuries[89]

Translator's Note: This chapter is extracted from Volume 13 of 《 驗方 新編 》 *Yàn Fāng Xīn Biān*. An additional section is included from 《 急救 易知 》 *Jí Jiù Yì Zhī* (Easily Understood Emergency Treatment): on treating a dislocated jaw.

損傷諸方 *Sǔn Shāng Zhū Fāng*
Various Formulas for Injury

回生第一仙丹 *Huí Shēng Dì Yī Xiān Dān*
(Most Effective Elixir of the Immortals for Returning Life)

治跌傷、壓傷、打傷、刀傷、銃傷、割喉、弔死、驚死、溺 水死等症（ 雷擊死雖未試過，想亦可治 ）。雖遍體重傷，死 已數日，祇要身體稍頓 。

This treats patterns such as injuries from falling, crushing, beatings, knives, guns, cutting the throat, hangings, death due to fright, and drowning. Even if there are severe injuries all over the whole body and the victim has already been dead for several days, it is only necessary that the body remains somewhat soft.

---

89. 跌打損傷 *diē dǎ sǔn shāng* literally means *injury from a fall or beating*. However, a functional translation is the more general *traumatic injuries*.

用此丹灌服，少刻即有微氣，再服一次，即活。大便如下紫血，更妙。惟身體殭硬者難救。

Pour this elixir into the patient. A moment later there will be slight qì [breath]. He will come back to life when he takes it one more time. If it looks like there is purple blood in the stool, this is even more wonderful. It is only difficult to rescue someone if his body is a hard stiff corpse.

此系豫章彭竹樓民部家傳秘方。道光初年，民部宰直隸時，有人被毆死已三日矣，民部往驗，見其肢體尚軟，打開一齒，以此丹灌服一分五厘，少刻其尸微動，再灌一分五厘而活。

This is a secret formula passed down in the family of Péng Zhúlóu of Yùzhāng, who was the Minister of Revenue. In 1821 (the first year of Dàoguāng's reign) at the time of the slaughter in Zhílì Province, the Minister of Revenue came upon someone who had been beaten and left for dead for three days earlier. The Minister of Revenue observed that the limbs and trunk were still soft. He broke open a tooth in order to pour in 1.5 *fēn* of this elixir and the corpse moved a moment later. He poured in another 1.5 *fēn* and the victim came back to life.

惟時磁州地震，壓斃甚眾，民部製丹遣人馳往，救活不下千人。

At the time of the Cízhōu earthquake when a great many people were crushed to death, the Minister of Revenue manufactured the elixir and sent people galloping toward the affected area with it. They rescued at least a thousand people.

活土鼈蟲（又名地鼈、又名簸箕蟲。形扁不能飛，大小不等，色黑而亮，背有橫楞，輪前窄後寬。以大如大指頭為佳；小者功緩。雄者更好；用刀截兩節放地上，以碗蓋住，過夜，其蟲自接而活，方是雄的。隨處皆有，多生米店有糠之處及碓臼下、倉底、竈腳，冬天竈腳更多，或生麪鋪，或油榨坊、並空屋乾燥之處，總在鬆土內尋覓。以活者，去足，放瓦上，小火焙黃，研細，用淨末五錢）。

Live *tŭ biē chóng*: It is also called *dì biē* (Earth Soft-Shelled Turtle), or *bò ji chóng* (Dustpan Bug). Its body is flat, it cannot fly, and it comes in different sizes. It is black and shiny with horizontal ridges on the back. It is round but the front is narrow and the back is wide. The big ones are the size of the end of the thumb and are good, but the small ones are slow to give results. Males are better. Cut one into two sections with a knife, place it on the ground, and cover it tightly with a bowl. If the bug reconnects itself over night and lives, it is male. They can be found everywhere. A lot live in shops that sell rice, where there is chaff and under the mortar and pestle, below the storehouse, or under the legs of the stove. There are even more under the legs of the stove during the winter. Some live in noodle shops, some in oil-press workshops, as well as in vacant rooms and dry places. In general, look for them inside loose soil. Remove the legs from live ones. Place them on a tile and stone-bake them over a low fire until yellow. Grind them finely and use five *qián* of clean powder.

自然銅（放瓦上木炭火內燒紅，入好醋內淬，半刻取出再燒再淬，連製九次，研末。要親身自；製藥店內製多不透不效。用淨末三錢）。

Zì rán tóng: Put it on a tile inside a charcoal fire and roast it until red. Quench it in good vinegar. After half of a quarter hour,[90] take it out, roast it and quench it again. Continuously prepare it this way for a total of nine times. Grind it into a powder. It is important to personally prepare it yourself. Often, what is prepared inside the pharmacy does not penetrate and is not effective. Use three *qián* of the clean powder.

真乳香（以形如乳頭黃色如膠者，為真；不真不效。每壹兩用燈草二錢五分同炒枯，與燈草同研細，吹去燈草得淨末，二錢）。

Genuine *rŭ xiāng*: The genuine is nipple-shaped, yellow, and glue-like.[91] If it is

---

90. It is not clear if this refers to half of a quarter Western single-hour (which would be 7.5 minutes) or half of a quarter Chinese double-hour (fifteen minutes).

91. The 乳 *rŭ* in 乳香 *rŭ xiāng* means breast or nipple so if it is nipple-shaped, its form agrees with its name. 膠 *jiāo* is translated as glue for lack of a better word. This is the same word as in 阿膠 *ē jiāo* and is the animal-product type of glue or gelatin. This is only its appearance, however; 乳香 *rŭ xiāng* comes

not genuine, it is not effective. Stir-fry each *liǎng* with 2.5 *qián* of *dēng cǎo* until dried out. Finely grind it along with the *dēng cǎo*. Blow on it to remove the *dēng cǎo* and thereby obtain a clean powder. Use two *qián*.

真陳血竭（ 飛淨，二錢 ）。真珠砂（ 飛淨，二錢 ）。巴豆
（ 去殼，研，用紙包壓數次去淨油，用淨末，二錢 ）。真麝
香（ 三分，要當門子 ）。

Genuine aged *xuè jié*: water grind and clean, two *qián*. Genuine *zhū shā*: water grind and clean, two *qián*. *Bā dòu*: remove the husk, grind, wrap in paper and press several times to remove the oil, use two *qián* of clean powder. Genuine *shè xiāng*: three *fēn*, it is important to use *dāng mén zǐ*.[92]

右藥揀選明淨，研極細末，收入小口磁瓶，用蠟封口，不可
洩氣 。大人每用一分五釐，小兒七釐 。酒沖服 。牙關不開
者，灌之必活 。

For the above, select medicinals that are bright and clean. Grind them into an extremely fine powder, and store it in a small-mouth porcelain bottle. Seal the opening with wax. It cannot leak qì [must be airtight]. Use one *fēn* five *lí* each time for adults. Use seven *lí* for children. Drench it in liquor and have the patient take it. If the jaw cannot open, pour it in and the patient will live.

活後，宜避風調養，若傷後受凍而死，須放煖室中，最忌見
火 。仍照急救門凍死法糸酌治之 。如活轉心腹疼痛；此瘀血
未淨，服白糖飲，自愈 。

After being revived, the patient should avoid wind and take good care of himself. If he is exposed to cold after the injury, he will die. He must stay inside a warm room. He should especially avoid exposure to fire. Consider treating it according to the method in the emergency treatment section on freezing to death. If it changes to pain in the heart region and abdomen when he is revived, the blood stasis is not yet cleaned out. He will automatically recover if he takes 白糖飲 *Bái Táng Yǐn* (White Sugar Drink) [see below].[93]

---

from the sap of a tree.

92. 當門子 *dāng mén zǐ* is a type of 麝香 *shè xiāng*, considered high quality.

93. On p. 117.

玉真散 *Yù Zhēn Sàn*
True Jade Powder

治跌打損傷已破口者，無論傷口大小，不省人事，或傷口潰
爛進風，口眼喎斜，手足扯動，形如彎弓，只要心前微溫，
用此藥敷傷口。（如膿多者，用溫茶避風洗淨再敷；無膿不
必洗）另用熱酒沖服三錢；不飲酒者滾水沖服，亦能起死回
生。惟嘔吐者難治。藥雖平淡，效最神奇，功在七釐、鐵扇
諸方之上，藥料易覓無假，其價亦廉。

This treats traumatic injuries from a fall or beating with open wounds. It doesn't
matter if the wound is large or small or the patient is unconscious. In some
the wound festers and wind enters, with deviation of the mouth and eyes.
The hands and feet pull and stir making the body arch like a drawn bow. So
long as there is slight warmth in front of the heart, apply this medicine to the
wound. (If there is a lot of pus, wash it clean with warm tea and then apply the
medicine; avoiding the wind. If there is no pus, you must not wash it.) Others
drench three *qián* of the powder in hot liquor and have the patient take it. If
someone does not drink liquor, drench it in boiling water and have the patient
take it. It is still able to raise the dead and return them to life. It is only difficult
to treat those who are vomiting. Even though the herbs in this formula are
ordinary, their effect is most miraculous and extraordinary. Its achievement is
superior to various formulas such as *Qī Lí Sàn* (Seven Lí Powder) or *Tiě Shàn
Sàn* (Iron Fan Powder).[94] The medicinal materials are easy to find without fakes
or substitutions. They are also inexpensive.

明天麻、羌活、防風、生南星（薑汁炒）、白芷（各一兩）
、白附子（十二兩）。右藥料須揀選明淨，研極細末，收入
小口磁瓶，以蠟封口，不可洩氣，如濕爛不能收口。用熟石
膏（二錢）、黃丹（二分）。共研極細，加入敷之。

---

94. 七釐散 *Qī Lí Sàn* (Seven Lí Powder) includes medicinal such as *zhū shā*
which are no longer considered acceptable for internal use. 鐵扇散 *Tiě Shàn
Sàn* (Iron Fan Powder) is another formula to treat open wounds. It contains
many obscure or unavailable medicinal, such as elephant skin, so these formulas will not be further described here.

Míng tiān má, qiāng huó, fáng fēng, shēng nán xīng (stir-fried in ginger juice), *bái zhǐ* (one *liǎng* of each); *bái fù zǐ* (twelve *liǎng*). When you select the above medicinal substances, they must be bright and clean. Grind them into an extremely fine powder, and store it in a small-mouth porcelain bottle. Seal the opening with wax. It cannot leak qì [must be airtight]. If it gets damp and sodden, it cannot close wounds. [At the time of use] grind *shú shí gāo* (two *qián*) and *huáng dān* (two *fēn*) together into an extremely fine powder. Add it in and apply it.

當歸湯 *Dāng Guī Tāng*
Dāng Guī Decoction

治跌打損傷未破口者，功能散瘀活血，雖已氣絕，灌之亦活。

Treats traumatic injuries from a fall or beating without open wounds. Its function is to scatter stasis and enliven the blood. Even if qì has already expired, he will still live when you pour it in.

當歸、澤瀉（各五錢）、川芎、紅花、桃仁、丹皮（各三錢）、好蘇木（二錢）。

dāng guī	當歸	5 *qián*
zé xiè	澤瀉	5 *qián*
chuān xiōng	川芎	3 *qián*
hóng huā	紅花	3 *qián*
táo rén	桃仁	3 *qián*
dān pí	丹皮	3 *qián*
good quality *sū mù*	蘇木	2 *qián*

右酒水各一碗，煎六分服。頭傷加藁本（一錢）；手傷加桂枝（一錢）；腰傷加杜仲（一錢）；脅傷加白芥子（一錢）；腳傷加牛膝（一錢）。

Place the above in one bowl each of liquor and water, boil until sixty percent, and have the patient take it.

- For injury to the head, add *gǎo běn* (one *qián*).
- For injury to the hands, add *guì zhī* (one *qián*).
- For injury to the low back, add *dù zhòng* (one *qián*).
- For injury to the rib-sides, add *bái jiè zǐ* (one *qián*).
- For injury to the legs, add *niú xī* (one *qián*).

白糖飲 *Bái Táng Yǐn*
White Sugar Drink

凡跌打損傷，如已氣絕，牙關緊閉。先用半夏在兩腮邊擦
之，牙關自開。急用熱酒沖白沙糖二三兩灌入；不飲酒者，
水服亦可。愈多愈妙，無論受傷輕重，服之可免瘀血攻心。

Whenever qì has already expired in traumatic injuries from a fall or beating, the jaw is tightly clenched. First rub *bàn xià* on the sides of the two cheeks, and the jaw will automatically open. Quickly drench two or three *liǎng* of white granulated sugar with hot liquor and pour it in. If the person does not drink liquor, he can also take it with water. The more he takes, the more wonderful it is. It doesn't matter if the injury is light or serious, taking this can avert static blood from attacking the heart.

又方：如氣絕不省人事，急用生半夏研末，水調黃豆大，塞
鼻孔，立能蘇醒，男左女右。醒後鼻痛，用老薑汁搽過，即
不痛也。

Another formula: If qì has expired and the person is unconscious, quickly grind *shēng bàn xià* into a powder. Mix it with water and [make a pellet] the size of a soybean, then stop up a nostril with it. He will immediately regain consciousness. Use the left nostril on males and the right on females. After regaining consciousness, his nose will hurt, [but] it will not hurt anymore after rubbing in juice from old ginger.

又方：野菊花連根陰乾，每用一兩，加酒與童便，各一碗煎
服，但有一絲之氣，無不活也。

Another formula: *yě jú huā* including the roots, dried in the shade. Use one *liǎng* each time. Add one bowl each of liquor and child's urine (*tóng biàn*), boil

117

and have the patient take it. If there is still any trace of qì, they will all recover.

又方：仙桃草，連根陰乾，研末，每服一二錢，開水送下。
雖傷重垂危，服之立效。

Another formula: *xiān táo cǎo* including the roots, dried in the shade. Grind it into a powder. Have the patient take one or two *qián* each time, swallowed down with boiled water. Even if it is a serious injury or a critical case, taking this is immediately effective.

江南一盜，身受多傷，躺臥道旁，一人路過見而憐之，村中
乞水與飲，盜出此藥調水服下，服後半刻，遍身傷處作響，
立即起而行矣。

A robber in Jiāngnán received a lot of damage [from a beating] and was lying by the side of the road. Someone passing down the road saw him and pitied him. In the village, he asked for some water and gave it to him to drink. The robber took out this medicine, mixed it with the water, and took it. Half a quarter hour after taking it, all the damaged sites on his body made sounds; he immediately got up and walked away.

詢之，此草生麥地中，葉小根紅，有子如胡椒大，內有一
蟲，在小暑節內前後採之。早則蟲尚未生；遲則蟲已飛去，
無蟲則無功效。聞廣西陽朔一帶亦有這種名麥杆草，八九月
內方有蟲生可采。

The other man asked about it and found that this herb grows in wheat fields. The leaves are small and the roots are red. It has seeds the size of *hú jiāo*. There is a bug inside. Gather it around the time of *xiǎo shǔ jié*.[95] If too early, the bug is not alive yet. If too late, the bug has already flown away. It is ineffective without the bug. I have heard that this species is also in the Yángshuò region of Guǎngxī province, where it is called *mài gān cǎo*; it can be picked in the eighth and ninth month when it has the live bug.

---

95. 小暑節 *xiǎo shǔ jié* (Slight Heat Solar Term) is the 11th Solar Term in the Chinese calendar (using the 二十四節氣 twenty-four *jié qì*). It takes place from around July 7th until July 21st in the northern hemisphere.

跌壓傷死 *Diē Yā Shāng Sǐ*
Death from Falls and Crushing Injuries

凡跌壓傷重之人，口耳出血，昏暈不醒，祇須身體尚頓，皆
可救活。切忌人多嘈雜，祇令家人呼而扶之。且就坐於地，
緊為抱定，曲其手足，如和尚打坐樣。隨以白糖沖熱酒灌之
（用水調灌亦可），尤為神妙。但能強灌一二杯下喉，便
好。

Whenever a person is seriously injured by falling or being crushed, he bleeds
from the mouth and ears. He faints and is unconscious. It is only important that
the body is still soft; all these cases can be resuscitated. By all means, avoid hav-
ing many noisy people around. Only let the family members cry out and help
him. For the time being just sit him down on the ground and hold on to him
firmly. Bend his hands and feet so he has the appearance of a Buddhist monk
sitting in meditation. Then drench white sugar with hot liquor and pour it into
him. (You can also mix it with water and pour it into him.) This is especially
marvelous; if you can force one or two cups of it down his throat, this is better.

然後抱入室內。如前坐法，更以足緊抵肛門；若係婦女，連
陰戶一並頂住；恐其氣從下洩，以致不救。並將窗櫺遮住，
以房中黑暗為佳。

After that, carry the patient into the house. If you used the above sitting
method, continue using his feet to tightly support his anus. If this is a woman,
support her yīn door [vagina] as well. Otherwise, the qì will leak out from
below and the patient cannot be rescued. At the same time, cover the windows.
It is good to make the inside of the room dark.

一面查照前後各方；取簡便者用之。傷重者瘀血必多，用前
當歸湯、白糖飲最妙。其餘簡便易得者，不妨兼用。

At the same time, refer to the formulas above and below. Select what is at hand
and use it. If the injury is serious, there will be a lot of blood stasis; using the
above *Dāng Guī Tāng* and *Bái Táng Yǐn* is most wonderful. You might as well
simultaneously use the others that are handy and easily obtained.

119

急切不可令出大便；恐其氣脫而死。必俟其腹中動而有聲，
上下往來數遍，急不能待，方可使解，所下盡是紫血。毒已
解下，方可令睡。倘瘀血未盡，當歸湯、白糖飲，尤宜多
服。

It is imperative that the patient is prevented from defecating. Otherwise his qì will desert and he will die. Wait for movement and sounds in his abdomen, up and down, going and coming several times. When it is urgent and he cannot wait, he can relieve himself. What is discharged will be full of purple blood. After the toxins have been discharged [with the stool], you can let the patient sleep. If the blood stasis is not entirely gone, he should especially take a lot of *Dāng Guī Tāng* and *Bái Táng Yǐn*.

又一切撲折，及從高墜下、木石傾壓、落馬、墜車，以致瘀
血凝滯氣絕欲死者。倉卒無藥，急以白糖服之。再取地上三
尺下黃土數升，搗碎，甑蒸熱，舊布重包，二包輪流熨傷
處，數次，痛止傷消，但不可太熱，恐傷皮肉。

Also, all falls that result in breaks, as well as tumbling from high places, crushing from collapsed wood or stone, falling from a horse, run over by a cart – these result in blood stasis congealing and stagnating, and qì expiring to the point of death. If you are in a hurry and do not have medicine, quickly have the patient take white sugar. Also gather several *shēng* of yellow earth (*huáng tǔ*, loess) from three *chǐ* under the surface. Crush and steam it in a rice pot. Wrap it in two layers of old cloth. Iron the injured site alternating the two bags. After several times, the pain will stop and the injury will disperse. However, it cannot be too hot or else it will damage the skin and flesh.

破口傷 *Pò Kǒu Shāng*
Open Wounds

龍眼核，剝去光皮不用，將核研極細，摻瘡口即定痛止血；
此西秦巴里坤營中急救方也，大有功效。如口渴者，不可飲
水，但食油膩之物以解其渴；更忌食粥，食則血必湧出而
死。或用前玉真散最妙。

Lóng yăn hé, peel the shiny skin off the pit and do not use it. Grind the pits into an extremely fine powder. When you sprinkle it onto the opening of the sore, it settles pain and stops bleeding. This was an emergency formula used in the *Bā Lǐ Kūn* camp of Western *Qín*.[96] It is very effective. If thirsty, the patient cannot drink water but can eat oily greasy things to resolve the thirst. Furthermore, he should avoid eating congee; when eaten, blood gushes out and the patient will die. Sometimes it is most effective to use the above formula *Yù Zhēn Sàn*.

又方：魚子蘭葉（珠蘭葉更好），搗融，敷之，立刻收口接骨。傷口寬大者，加白鹽少許，第二次敷，即不用鹽，其效非常，功在諸方之上。

Another formula: *yú zī lán yè* (*zhū lán yè* is even better). Pound it until soft and apply it. It immediately closes the opening and joins bones. If the opening of the wound is wide and big, add a little white salt. Do not use salt in the second application. The effect is extraordinary. Its achievement is superior to all other formulas.

又方：月季花（又名月月紅），取葉搗爛，敷之，立能止血消腫，雖斷筋，亦可速愈。

Another formula: *yuè jì huā* (also called *yuè yuè hóng*). Pound the leaves into a pulp and apply it. It can immediately stop bleeding and disperse swelling. Even if a sinew is severed, it can still heal quickly.

又方：葱白、沙糖等分，搗爛，研如泥，敷傷口，其疼立止，又無疤痕，屢試神驗。

Another formula: Equal portions of *cōng bái* and granulated sugar. Pound them into a pulp. Grind it until it is the consistency of mud and apply it to the wound. The pain will immediately stop. It also will not leave a scar. This has been tried repeatedly and gives miraculous experiences.

---

96. 西秦 *Xī qín* Western *Qín* was one of the Sixteen Kingdoms, one of the sixteen northern states during the *Jìn* dynasty (385-431). 巴里坤 *Bā Lǐ Kūn* refers to Barkol Kazakh autonomous county or Barköl Qazaq aptonom nahiyisi in Kumul prefecture, *Xīnjiāng*.

又方：生半夏研末敷上，即刻止痛，且易收口 。

Another formula: Grind *shēng bàn xià* into a powder and apply it to the wound. It will stop the pain at once; furthermore it allows the opening to close easily.

又方：生松香，熟松香，和勻敷之，立愈，或加生半夏末亦可 。此軍營急救方也 。

Another formula: Blend fresh and cooked *sōng xiāng* evenly and apply it. The wound will immediately recover. *Shēng bàn xià* powder can also be added. This is an emergency prescription from the military.

又方：老薑嚼融敷之，數日平複如常，此方屢試屢驗，可保不致進風 。惟敷時痛極，忍耐幾時可耳 。

Another formula: Chew old ginger until soft and apply it. In several days [the wound] will be level and returned to normal. This formula has been repeatedly tried and is repeatedly effective. It can prevent progression of wind [in the wound]. The pain is extreme only at the time of application and must be endured for a few hours.

又方：胡椒末敷之，不惟速愈，且免縮筋，忍痛必效 。

Another formula: Apply powdered *hú jiāo* to it. This not only brings speedy recovery, it is certainly effective for preventing contraction of the sinews and the suffering of pain.

止血法 *Zhǐ Xuè Fǎ*
Methods to Stop Bleeding

瘦豬肉切濃片貼上，無論傷口大小、血流不止者，立效如神 。或用豬皮亦可 。此急救止血第一方也 。

Apply a think slice of lean pork on top, regardless of the size of the wound, even if it won't stop bleeding; it is immediately miraculously effective. You can also use pork skin. This is the best emergency formula to stop bleeding.

122

又方：草紙燒灰，候冷敷上亦止。

Another formula: Burn rice paper to ash, wait until it cools, and apply the ash on top; this also stops bleeding.

又方：老薑燒枯存性，研末敷，亦神效也。

Another formula: Roast old ginger until dried up, preserving its nature.[97] Grind it into a powder and apply it. This is also miraculously effective.

跌打吐血不止 *Diē Dǎ Tǔ Xiě Bù Zhǐ*
Incessant Vomiting of Blood after Trauma such as a Fall or Beating

荷花焙乾，研末，酒調服，一日二三次，數日即愈，其效如神。乾荷葉亦可，或多服白糖飲更妙。

Stone-bake *hé huā* until dry, and grind them into powder. Mix with liquor and have the patient take it once or twice a day. He will recover after several days. The effect is miraculous! You can also use dried *hé yè*. Or taking a lot of *Bái Táng Yǐn* is even more wonderful.

破口傷風 *Pò Kǒu Shāng Fēng*
Wind in an Open Wound

凡破傷風寒熱交作，口閉咬牙，或吐白沫，手足扯動，或頭足扯如彎弓，傷口平塌者，最為險症。用前玉真散，可以起死回生，最為神妙。

Whenever there is tetanus (*pò shāng fēng*), there will be simultaneous [aversion to] cold and heat. The mouth clenches shut. Some spit frothy saliva. The arms and legs pull and stir. Sometimes the head and feet pull until the back is arched like a drawn bow. The most critical symptoms occur when the wound becomes flat or sunken [rather than swollen]. Use the above *Yù Zhēn Sàn*. It can raise the dead and return them to life. It is the most miraculous wonder!

---

97. 'Preserving its nature' means that the original properties are still present, so it is not charred to a crisp.

如倉卒製藥不及，用手指甲腳趾甲各一錢，香油炒黃，研末，熱酒調服，汗出即愈。終不如玉真散之妙。

If in a hurry to make medicine, while inferior, you can use one *qián* each of fingernails and toenails. Stir-fry them in sesame oil until yellow, and grind them into a powder. Mix with hot liquor and have the patient take it. He will recover after sweating. In the end, this is not as good as the wonderful *Yù Zhēn Sàn*.

下頦脫落 *Xià Hái Tuō Luò*
Dislocation of the Jaw[98]

此症起於腎肺虛損，元神不足，或談笑高興忘倦，一時元氣不能接續所致。

This pattern arises in kidney-lung vacuity detriment and insufficiency of original spirit. This is perhaps caused by someone talking and laughing, happy, forgetting fatigue; in a short while, original qì cannot join [sinew and bone].

須平身正坐，令人以兩手托住下頦，向腦後送上關竅，隨用布條兜住。務須避風；若受風邪，痰涎上壅，口眼歪，邪則難治矣。

The patient must sit straight with his body level. Make someone hold his lower jaw with both hands and deliver it toward the back of the head into the socket of the upper joint of the jaw. Then bind it in place with a strip of cloth. The patient must avoid wind; if he contracts wind evils, phlegm-drool will congest in the upper body, the mouth and eyes will deviate, and these evils will be difficult to treat.

外用天南星研末，薑汁調敷兩腮頰，一夜即上。次日再用：高麗參、白術、茯苓、製半夏（各五錢）、當歸（二錢）、僵蚕（二錢）、天麻、陳皮（各一錢）、川芎（八分）、甘草（三分）、製附子（六分）、燈心（十四根）、生薑（三片）。

---

98. This section is not in《驗方新編》*Yàn Fāng Xīn Biān* (New Compilation of Proven Formulas), but was taken from《急救易知》*Jí Jiù Yì Zhī* (Easily Understood Emergency Treatment).

Externally, mix powdered *tiān nán xīng* with ginger juice and apply it to both cheeks. The jaw will ascend into place overnight. Then the next day use:

gāo lí shēn	高麗參	5 *qián*
bái zhú	白尤	5 *qián*
fú líng	茯苓	5 *qián*
zhì bàn xià	製半夏	5 *qián*
dāng guī	當歸	2 *qián*
jiāng cán	僵蚕	2 *qián*
tiān má	天麻	1 *qián*
chén pí	陳皮	1 *qián*
chuān xiōng	川芎	8 *fēn*
gān cǎo	甘草	3 *fēn*
zhì fù zǐ	製附子	6 *fēn*
dēng xīn	燈心	14 strands
shēng jiāng	生薑	3 slices

右水煎服 。

Boil the above in water and have the patient take it internally.

又方：真烏梅搗融為餅，塞滿牙盡頭處，張口流涎，隨手掇
上 。

Another formula: Genuine *wū méi* pounded soft and made into a cake. Stuff it into the place at the end of the teeth. Open the mouth, let saliva flow, and put the jaw up in place without trouble.

又方：白尤（ 一兩 ）、防風（ 五錢 ）。右水煎服，半刻即
上，其效甚速 。

Another formula: Boil *bái zhú* (one *liǎng*) and *fáng fēng* (five *qián*) in water and have the patient take it internally. In half a quarter hour,[99] the jaw will go back up. The effect is extremely rapid.

---

99. It is not clear if this refers to half of a quarter Western single-hour (which would be 7.5 minutes) or half of a quarter Chinese double-hour (fifteen minutes).

割頸斷喉 *Gē Jǐng Duàn Hóu*
Cut Neck or Severed Throat

急宜早救；遲則額冷氣絕，乘初割時，輕輕扶住，使仰睡，
將頭墊起，合攏刀口，將血拭去。用生松香、熟松香各半，
或加生半夏末亦可，將傷口厚厚敷緊。（或用蔥頭和白蜜，
搗融敷，亦可。）外用膏藥（不論何項膏藥），周圍連好
肉，一併黏貼，再用布條圍裹，鉤線縫好。

It is urgent that you try to rescue this patient early; when you are late, the
forehead is cold and qì has expired, so make the most of the initial time when
the throat was cut. Lightly and gently support the victim and let him lie down
face up. Raise his head with a cushion. Close up the incision and wipe away
the blood. Use equal portions of fresh *sōng xiāng* and cooked *sōng xiāng*. You
can also add *shēng bàn xià* powder. Apply a very thick layer of it to seal up the
wound. (*Cōng tóu* can also be blended with white honey, pounded until soft,
and applied.) On the outside of this, stick a medicated plaster (it doesn't matter
which medicated plaster) onto the good flesh, surrounding the wound and the
other glue [meaning the *sōng xiāng*]. Then bind it with a piece of cloth and sew
it up securely with thread.

每日服玉真散（三錢），覺傷處生肌，即不必服，未生肌，
則日日常服。無論食嗓氣嗓俱斷，一月必愈，屢試如神。若
食氣嗓俱未斷，照前傷損各方治之，亦可如氣嗓已斷，祇須
身體微輭。一面照前敷治，一面以回生丹服之，亦可活也。

Every day the patient should take three *qián* of *Yù Zhēn Sàn*, but when you find
that the wound is regenerating flesh, he must stop taking it. Before the wound
regenerates flesh, have the patient take this formula constantly every day. Regardless of whether the esophagus and trachea are both severed, he will recover
in one month. This has been repeatedly tested and it works like a miracle! If
neither the esophagus nor the trachea are severed, treat it according to the
above trauma formulas. You can treat it as if the trachea had been severed only
if the body is still slightly soft. On the one hand, treat it according to the above
application method (using *sōng xiāng*); on the other hand, have the patient

take *Huí Shēng Dān* (Return to Life Elixir).[100] Then he can still live.

戳傷腸出 *Chuō Shāng Cháng Chū*
The Intestines Come Out After a Stabbing

好醋煮熱洗之（不可太熱，亦不可冷），隨洗隨入。外用活剝雞皮，乘熱貼上。再服玉真散，自愈。愈後雞皮自落。

Wash [the wound including the intestines] with good vinegar that has been boiled hot (it cannot be too hot; it also cannot be cold). After washing, put the intestines back in. Externally stick on skin flayed from a live chicken while it is still hot. Then have the patient take *Yù Zhēn Sàn* for automatic recovery. After recovery, the chicken skin will automatically fall off.

手指砍斷 *Shǒu Zhǐ Kǎn Duàn*
Severed Fingers

將指接上，用蘇木細末敷之。外用蠶繭包縛牢固，數日即愈。

To reconnect a finger, apply finely powdered *sū mù* to it. Externally wrap and bind it firmly with silkworm cocoon (*cán jiǎn*). It will recover in several days.

又方：老薑嚼融敷之，新棉包裹，簡便神效。

Another formula: Chew old ginger until soft, apply it, and wrap [the wound] up in new cotton. This is simple, convenient, and miraculously effective.

---

100. 回生丹 *Huí Shēng Dān* (Return to Life Elixir) is the first formula in this chapter. The full name is 回生第一仙丹 *Huí Shēng Dì Yī Xiān Dān* (Most Effective Elixir of the Immortals for Returning Life).

接骨法 *Jiē Gú Fǎ*
Method for Setting Bones

杉木炭，研極細末，用白沙糖蒸極融化，將炭末和勻，攤紙
上，乘熱貼之，無論破骨、傷筋、斷指、折足，數日可愈，
屢試屢驗。忌食生冷發物。無杉木炭，用杉木燒枯亦可。

Grind *shān mù tàn*[101] into an extremely fine powder. Steam white granulated sugar until completely melted and blend evenly with the charcoal powder. Spread the mixture on paper and stick the plaster on while it is still hot. It doesn't matter if a bone is broken, a sinew is injured, a finger is severed, or a leg is broken – the patient can recover in several days. This has been repeatedly tested through repeated experience. Avoid eating fresh cold or stimulating foods. If you don't have *shān mù tàn*, you can substitute *shān mù* that has been roasted until it is dried out.

又方：凡骨斷痛極者，先用鳳仙花根（一寸，以肥大者為
佳），磨酒服之，操動不痛。然後可用藥治。或用麻藥敷
之，亦不痛也。

Another formula: Whenever bones are severed, the pain is extreme. First grind up *fèng xiān huā gēn* (one *cùn* long, fat large ones are good). The patient should take it with liquor. Then he can move without pain. Afterwards you can treat it with [other] medicine. Some also apply numbing medicine [anesthetic] to it so that it is not painful.

又方：當歸（七錢五分）、川芎（五錢）、乳香、沒藥（各
式錢半）、木香（一錢）、川烏（四錢五分）、黃丹（六
錢）、骨碎補（五錢）、古錢（照前製法[102]，三錢）。

Another formula:

dāng guī	當歸	7.5 *qián*
chuān xiōng	川芎	5 *qián*

---

101. Charcoal from Chinese fir wood.
102. The Chinese text says "the method above" but the directions are actually given below.

rǔ xiāng	乳香		2.5 *qián*
mò yào	沒藥		2.5 *qián*
mù xiāng	木香		1 *qián*
chuān wū	川烏		4.5 *qián*
huáng dān	黃丹		6 *qián*
gǔ suì bǔ	骨碎補		5 *qián*
gǔ qián	古錢	processed according to the method below.	3 coins

右共為細末，入香油一兩五錢，調成膏，貼患處。雖骨碎筋斷，能續，神效。

Finely powder the above together. Put it in 1.5 *liǎng* of sesame oil. Mix it into an ointment and stick it onto the affected site. Even if the bone is shattered and the sinews are severed, they can reconnect. It is miraculously effective.

又方：古銅錢燒紅，淬入好醋內，再燒再淬，連製七次，研末，用酒沖服二錢，傷大者服三錢，其骨自接。無古銅錢，用新銅錢亦可，不如古銅錢之妙。

Another formula: Heat ancient copper coins until red hot and quench them in good vinegar. Repeat the heating and quenching a total of seven times, and then grind them into a powder. Drench two *qián* in alcohol and take it; if the damage is great, take three *qián*. The bones will automatically join. If you do not have ancient copper coins, new copper coins can also be used but they are not as wonderful as ancient copper coins.

跌打傷筋 *Diē Dǎ Shāng Jīn*
Damage to the Sinews from Trauma such as a Fall or Beating

用韭菜搗爛敷，過一夜即愈。

Pound *jiǔ cài* into a pulp and apply it to recover after leaving it on for one night.

又方：生旋覆花根，搗汁滴入，並敷。日換三次，至半月。雖筋斷，亦續，其效如神。

Another formula: Crush *shēng xuán fù huā gēn* to extract the juice and drip it on. At the same time apply it to the affected site. Change it three times a day for up to half a month. Even if the sinew is severed, it still can reconnect. Its effect is miraculous!

傷損縮筋年久不愈 *Shāng Sǔn Suō Jīn Nián Jiǔ Bù Yù*
Contraction of the Sinews that has Lasted for Years after an Injury without Recovery

楊梅樹皮，曬乾研末，和頂好燒酒，蒸熟調敷，用布紮好，每日一換，不過三五次。即愈，屢試如神，不可輕視。

Dry *yáng méi shù pí* in the sun and grind it into a powder. Blend with the best quality white distilled liquor (*shāo jiǔ*). Steam it until completely cooked, mix, and apply it. Bind it on securely with cloth. Change it once a day. The patient will recover in not more than three or five applications. This has been tested repeatedly and works like a miracle; you should not underestimate it.

腳趾割破久不收口行走不便
Jiǎo Zhǐ Gē Pò Jiǔ Bù Shōu Kǒu Háng Zǒu Bù Biàn
The Toes Cut Open without [the Wound] Closing Up for a Long Time, with Difficulty Walking

雞腳骨燒枯研末敷，即愈，甚效。

The patient will recover when chicken leg bones are roasted until dried out, ground into a powder, and applied. This is extremely effective.

跌打青腫 *Diē Dǎ Qīng Zhǒng*
Black and Blue[103] Swelling from Trauma such as a Fall or Beating

整塊生大黃，用生薑汁磨，濃敷之，一夜，紫者轉黑，黑者
即白矣，一日一換，其效如神。

Grind an entire piece of *shēng dà huáng* with ginger juice and apply a thick
layer of it. The purple will turn black overnight. The black will then turn white.
Change it once a day. The effect is miraculous!

又方：生半夏水調敷。一夜即消。

Another formula: Apply *shēng bàn xià* mixed with water. It will disperse overnight.

跌打青腫內傷 *Diē Dǎ Qīng Zhǒng Nèi Shāng*
Internal Damage with Black and Blue Swelling from
Trauma such as a Fall or a Beating

凡一切跌打損傷，遍身青腫，瘀停作痛，及墮仆內傷，一服
即愈。用白木耳四兩（如無白者，黑亦可用）焙乾，為細
末，服一兩，麻油拌勻，好酒送服，二次藥完，其患若失，
百發百中，神妙非常。

Whenever there are any traumatic injuries from a fall or a beating, the whole
body is black and blue and swollen. The collecting blood stasis is painful and
there is internal damage from falling down. The patient will recover as soon
as he takes *bái mù ěr* (the black can be substituted for the white). Stone-bake
four *liǎng* until dry, and make it into a fine powder. The patient should take one
liǎng mixed evenly with sesame oil, swallowed with good liquor. After finish-
ing the medicine twice, the suffering will seem to be lost. It will hit the mark a
hundred percent of the time. It is extraordinarily miraculous.

---

103. 青 *qīng* is most often translated as *green-blue* or *green*. However, in this
context, it is more akin to the phrase *black and blue* in English.

打傷眼睛 *Dǎ Shāng Yǎn Jīng*
Damage to the Eyes from a Beating

凡眼睛打出，或跌傷、碰傷、或火爆傷，用南瓜瓤搗爛，厚封。外用布包好勿動，漸即腫消痛定，乾則再換。如瞳人未破，仍能視也。瓜以愈老愈佳，有鮮地黃處，用地黃亦可。

Whenever an eye is punched out or injured from a fall, collision, or fiery explosion, use *nán guā ráng* pounded to a pulp. Seal [the eye socket] with a thick layer. On the outside wrap it securely with cloth and do not let the patient move. Gradually, the swelling will disperse and the pain will settle. Change it when it gets dry. If the pupil is not damaged, he will still be able to see. The older the melon, the better. If you are in a place that has *xiān dì huáng*, you can also use *dì huáng*.

又方：生豬肉一斤，以當歸、赤石脂二味研末，摻肉上貼之，拔出瘀血，眼即無恙。

Another formula: Grind *dāng guī* and *chì shí zhī* into a powder, sprinkle it on one *jīn* of fresh pork, and apply it. This draws out blood stasis so the eyes will be safe and sound.

閃跌手足 *Shǎn Diē Shǒu Zú*
Wrenching the Arms or Legs in a Fall

生薑、葱白、搗融，和灰麵炒熱，敷之。或用生大黃，和生薑汁磨敷，均妙。

Pound *shēng jiāng* and *cōng bái* until soft. Blend it with grey flour (*huī miàn*)[104] that has been stir-fried hot and apply it. Some grind *shēng dà huáng* blended with *shēng jiāng* juice and apply it. This is equally wonderful.

---

104. 灰麵 *huī miàn* (literally 'grey flour') is flour that is mixed with the juice of herbs, including 蓬柴草 *péng chái cáo*. This turns it grey, hence its name.

跌打損傷濕爛不乾 *Diē Dǎ Sǔn Shāng Shī Làn Bù Gān*
Traumatic Injuries that become
Damp Putrid Injuries and do not Dry Out

並治凍瘡濕爛。羊皮金紙，以金面貼傷處，過夜即愈，神效之至。

This equally treats damp and putrid frostbite sores. Stick the gold surface of gilded parchment[105] onto the wound. It will recover overnight and is miraculously effective to an extreme.

又方：寒水石二錢，煆研細末，敷之，立見功效。

Another formula: Calcine and grind *hán shuǐ shí* (two *qián*) into a fine powder and apply it. It has an immediate effect.

跌打損傷內有積血大小便不通
Diē Dǎ Sǔn Shāng Nèi Yǒu Jī Xiě Dà Xiǎo Biàn Bù Tōng
Traumatic Injuries from a Fall or Beating
Resulting in Internal Accumulation of Blood with
Inhibited Urination and Bowel Movement

歸尾（二錢）、生地、川芎、桃仁、生大黃、紅花
（各一錢）。

guī wěi	歸尾	2 *qián*
shēng dì	生地	1 *qián*
chuān xiōng	川芎	1 *qián*
táo rén	桃仁	1 *qián*
shēng dà huáng	生大黃	1 *qián*
hóng huā	紅花	1 *qián*

---

105. 羊皮金紙 *yáng pí jīn zhǐ*: This is parchment that is gilded on one side.

右酒水各半煎服；不飲酒者。無酒亦可。

Boil the above in equal amounts of liquor and water and have the patient take it. If the patient does not drink liquor, you can also make it without the liquor.

跌打損傷胸膈脹痛不食
Diē Dǎ Sǔn Shāng Xiōng Gé Zhàng Tòng Bù Shí
Traumatic Injuries from a Fall or a Beating with Distention and Pain in the Chest and Diaphragm, and Inability to Eat

白沙糖用酒沖服（ 水沖服亦可 ），以多為妙。

Drench white granulated sugar in liquor and give it to the patient (it can also be drenched in water and taken). Using a lot is wonderful.

舊傷日久作痛或天陰作痛
Jiù Shāng Rì Jiǔ Zuò Tòng Huò Tiān Yīn Zuò Tòng
Old Injuries that are Painful over the Course of Time or Painful in Cloudy Weather

益母草熬膏（ 忌鐵器 ），為丸，每服數錢，熱酒送下，十日全愈，其效如神。

Simmer *yì mǔ cǎo* into a paste (avoid ironware) and make it into a pill. The patient should take several *qián* per dose, swallowing it with hot liquor. Complete recovery will come in ten days. The effect is miraculous!

止血補傷方 *Zhǐ Xuè Bǔ Shāng Fāng*
Formula to Stop Bleeding and Mend Injuries

刀箭傷、馬踏傷、跌傷、一切物打傷均效。生白附子（ 十二兩 ）、白芷、天麻、生南星、防風、羌活（ 各一兩 ）。

This is equally effective for knife or arrow wounds, or injuries from being trampled by a horse, a fall, or being hit by something.

shēng bái fù zǐ	生白附子	12 *liǎng*
bái zhǐ	白芷	1 *liǎng*
tiān má	天麻	1 *liǎng*
shēng nán xīng	生南星	1 *liǎng*
fáng fēng	防風	1 *liǎng*
qiāng huó	羌活	1 *liǎng*

共研極細，就破處敷上。傷重者，用黃酒浸服數錢。青腫者，水調敷上。一切破爛，皆可敷之，即愈。此方宜平時預製，以治斗傷，可活兩命，價不昂而藥易得，亦莫大之陰功也。

Grind it all together into an extremely fine powder, and simply apply it to the broken site. If the damage is serious, soak the powder in yellow liquor and have the patient take several *qián* internally. If there is black and blue swelling, mix it with water and apply it. The patient will recover after applying it to any type of open wound or putrefaction. This formula should be prepared in normal times in order to treat injuries from fights; it can save two lives. It is not costly, the herbs are easy to obtain, and there is also no greater secret good deed.[106]

---

106. In the concept of karma, more merit is accumulated when good deeds are done in secret.

Chapter 8

刑杖傷 *Xíng Zhàng Shāng*
Injury from Flogging with a Cane

Translator's Note: This chapter is abridged from Volume 13 of 《驗方新編》*Yàn Fāng Xīn Biān*.

杖傷 *Zhàng Shāng*
Caning Injury

血竭（ 一錢 ）、輕粉、黃丹（ 水飛淨各二錢 ）、白礬（ 一錢 ）。

xuè jié	血竭		1 *qián*
qīng fěn	輕粉		2 *qián*
huáng dān	黃丹	water grind and clean	2 *qián*
bái fán	白礬		1 *qián*

右共為末，摻上，忍痛一時，次日其肉四圍生起，兩日即平。杖傷久爛不愈，中有深眼不能收口。用此最效。或照跌打損傷各方治之，亦可。

Powder the above together, and sprinkle it on the affected site. The patient must endure the pain for a while. The next day the flesh will grow in and rise up all around [the wound's depression caused by the caning]. In two days, the flesh will be level. Injuries from flogging with a cane can putrefy for a long time without recovering, with a deep opening in the center that does not close up.

This formula is the most effective. You can also treat it according to the various formulas for traumatic injuries from a fall or beating.

又方：杖後即飲童便一碗，或用酒沖白糖服之。不飲酒者，水服亦可，以免瘀血攻心。

Another formula: After the caning, drink a bowl of child's urine or drench white sugar with liquor and have the patient drink it. If he does not drink liquor, you can instead have him take it with water. This prevents static blood from attacking the heart.

再用熱豆腐鋪在杖傷處，其氣如蒸，其腐即紫，換腐數次，令紫色散盡，轉淡紅色為度。

Also spread hot tofu on the sites injured by the caning. Its qì seems like steam and turns the tofu purple. Change the tofu several times. Make the purple color dissipate completely. When the tofu turns light red, this is the degree [of success].

又受刑杖極重者，杖後日用白及末米湯飲下，神效。

Also, someone who received punishment by caning and is in extremely serious condition should swallow *bái jí* powder with rice soup every day after the caning. This has miraculous effects.

Chapter 9

銅鐵竹木雜物傷 *Tóng Tiě Zhú Mù Zá Wù Shāng*
Injury from Copper, Iron, Bamboo, Wood, and Miscellaneous Things

Translator's Note: This chapter is abridged from Volume 13 of 《驗方新編》 *Yàn Fāng Xīn Biān*, except the last two headings which come from 《急救易知》 *Jí Jiù Yì Zhī* (Easily Understood Emergency Treatment).

鐵鍼入肉 *Tiě Zhēn Rù Ròu*
An Iron Needle Embedded in the Flesh

針入肉內，隨氣游走，若走至心窩甚險。急用烏鴉翎數根，瓦上焙焦黃色，研細末，酒調服一錢。外用車輪上油垢，調真磁石末，攤紙上如錢大，貼之，每日一換，自出。

An iron needle embedded in the flesh wanders about following the qì. It is extremely dangerous if it arrives at the pit of the stomach. Quickly bake several crow feathers on a tile until burnt yellow, and grind it into powder. Mix it with liquor and take one *qián*. Externally mix the greasy dirt from the wheel of a cart with genuine *cí shí* (magnetite) powder. Spread it on paper, the size of a coin, and apply it, changing it once a day; the needle will automatically come out.

又方：生磁石（一錢）研末。用菜油調敷皮外離鍼入處寸許，漸漸移至鍼口，由受傷原處而出，神效。

Grind genuine *cí shí* (one *qián*) into a powder. Mix it with vegetable oil and apply it to the skin about a *cùn* away from the place where the needle entered. Little by little the needle will move through the needle hole and come out from the original site of the wound. It is miraculously effective.

鐵彈入肉 *Tiě Dàn Rù Ròu*
An Iron Bullet Embedded in the Flesh

扁魚肚膽（俗呼邊魚）煮融，和糯米飯，搗爛敷之，換兩三次，即出；此在手足及兩股用之。

Boil bream maw and gall bladder (*biǎn yú dù dǎn*, commonly called *biān yú*) until soft, and blend it with cooked glutinous rice. Pound it into a pulp and apply it. The bullet will come out when you have changed it two or three times. Use this method on the hands, feet, and the thighs.

若在身上及腹內，用土狗同扁魚肚，煮融搗爛敷，雖不能取出，其彈漸落下部，不能為害矣。

If the bullet is embedded in the body or inside the abdomen, use *tǔ gǒu* along with the bream maw (*biǎn yú dù*). Boil them until soft, pound them into a pulp, and apply it. Even if it is unable to extract it, the bullet will gradually drop to the lower parts where it is unable to do harm.

銅鐵礮子並一切雜物入肉
Tóng Tiě Pào Zǐ Bìng Yī Qiē Zá Wù Rù Ròu
Copper or Iron Cannon Shot and All Types of Miscellaneous Things Embedded in the Flesh

蜣螂（三箇）、巴豆（四五粒）。右共搗如泥，敷傷處，先止痛，後作癢，少刻，其物必出。

Pound *qiāng láng* (three of them) and *bā dòu* (four or five pieces) together until they are the consistency of mud, and apply it to the injured site. At first it stops the pain; afterwards it makes itching. A moment later, the object will come out.

又方：南瓜，搗融四圍敷之，隔日必出，極效 。

Another formula: Pound pumpkin until soft and apply it all around. It must be removed the following day. This is extremely effective.

又方：紅膏藥敷之，無不出 。

Another formula: Apply *Hóng Gāo Yào* (Red Plaster)[107] to it; it never fails to come out.

瓷片入肉 *Cí Piàn Rù Ròu*
A Porcelain Shard Embedded in the Flesh

白果（ 要三角形者，去壳與心 ）不拘多少，菜子油内，取出，搗融貼之，日換一次 。雖入肉多年，爛而不出者，三次，即愈 。

Bái guǒ (it is important to use the triangle-shaped kind, remove the shell and the core), the quantity is not limited. Remove the oil from the seeds. Mash them and stick it on. Change it once a day. Even if the shard has been inside the flesh for many years, putrefying without coming out, the patient will recover after three applications.

魚肉各骨入肉 *Yú Ròu Gè Gú Rù Ròu*
Various Types of Fish Bones Embedded in the Flesh

山楂研末調敷 。如在口中牙縫等處，山楂煎濃汁含一二時，自出 。

Grind *shān zhá* into a powder. Mix[108] and apply it. If the injury is in a place like the inside the mouth or between the teeth, boil *shān zhá* into a concentrated

---

107. 紅膏藥 *Hóng Gāo Yào* (Red Plaster) is found in Volume 11 of 《 驗方新編 》 *Yàn Fāng Xīn Biān*. See appendix on p. 198.

108. It seems there should be a liquid mentioned here, but one is not specified.

liquid and hold it in the mouth for one or two hours.[109] It will automatically come out.

竹木入肉 *Zhú Mù Rù Ròu*
Bamboo or Wood Embedded in the Flesh

鹿角（ 燒枯存性 ）研末 。以水調敷 。久不出者 。不過一夜 。
即出 。

Grind *lù jiǎo* (roasted until it is dried out, preserving its nature)[110] into a powder. Mix the powder with water and apply it. Even if the splinter has not come out for a long time, it will come out in not more than one night.

又方：松香敷上，用布包裹，三日必出，不痛不癢，甚妙 。

Another formula: Apply *sōng xiāng* on top of the site, and bind it with cloth. In three days the splinter will come out without pain or itching. This is extremely wonderful.

又方：生蒲公英搗敷 。雖腫爛日久，亦效 。

Another formula: Pound fresh *pú gōng yīng* and apply it. It is still effective even if there has been swelling and putrefaction for many days.

又方：鮮牛膝搗爛敷 。縱傷口已合，刺亦自出 。

Another formula: Pound fresh *niú xī* to a pulp and apply it. Even if the wound has already closed, the splinter will still automatically come out.

又方：萆麻子搗爛敷 。痛止，即出 。

Another formula: Pound *bì má zǐ* to a pulp and apply it. The splinter will come out when the pain stops.

---

109. It is not clear if this refers to two Western single-hours or two Chinese double-hours.

110. 'Preserving its nature' means that the original properties are still present, so it is not charred to a crisp.

水銀入肉 *Shuǐ Yín Rù Ròu*
Mercury in the Flesh

真川椒研末，生雞蛋白調敷，用布包緊，過夜即出 。

Grind genuine *chuān jiāo* into a powder. Mix it with fresh chicken egg whites and apply it. Wrap the affected site tightly with cloth. The mercury will come out over night.

針戳釀膿 *Zhēn Chuō Niàng Nóng*
A Needle Wound that Brews Pus

用煤炭擂末，白沙糖拌融敷 。雖腫痛釀膿者，亦效 。

Pestle coal (*méi tàn*) into a powder. Mix it with white sugar until soft and apply it. Even if it is swollen, painful, and brewing pus, this is still effective.

小兒誤將竹木刺入眼內
Xiǎo Ér Wù Jiāng Zhú Mù Cì Rù Yǎn Nèi
A Child Accidentally Sticks a Bamboo or Wood Splinter in the Eye

搗白梅如泥，罨之，即出 。瘡中胬肉同治 。

It will come out when you pound *bái méi* until it is the consistency of mud and use it as a compress. Treat outcroppings[111] in the sore the same way.

---

111. 胬肉 *nǔ ròu* (outcroppings): This is similar to the Western medical diagnosis of pterygium. Outcroppings can grow over the eye due to the irritation of the sore.

Chapter 10

蠱毒 *Gǔ Dú*
Gǔ Toxins[112]

Translator's Note: This is abridged from the chapter on *gǔ* toxins in Volume 15 of 《驗方新編》 *Yàn Fāng Xīn Biān*.

生蛇蠱 *Shēng Shé Gǔ*
Live Snake *Gǔ*

中其毒，或肚痛極、或作吐作瀉。自後凡遇肚痛時，行動則皮內或肚內有物堅實，夜臥以手按之，則肚皮內有物腫起，長二三寸，微覺跳動，心煩涎溢，得吃肉則止。或跳上心，則心脹欲作吐。又此物在身，時有時無，至四、五年則成形，會咬。又有變成肉鱉、肉龜以作咬者。至蛇老時在皮內、肚內行咬，有日咬二三十次者，命在頃刻。此時內蛇翻動作咬，則通身發熱，額焦、頭痛，如有發刺蟻咬，夜則更甚。此乃蠱家之外蛇從風而至也。內蛇咬臟腑，外蛇入毛孔，其蛇無形，亦無數。

When struck by these toxins, there may be severe pains in the belly, vomiting, or diarrhea. From then on, whenever there is pain in the belly, something solid moves around in the skin or the belly. At night when the patient presses it, something two or three *cùn* long swells up inside the skin or the belly and it can be felt to jump about slightly. There is also heart vexation and drool overflows.

---

112. 蠱 *gǔ*: The toxins of 蟲 *chóng* (bugs, reptiles, snakes, etc.) that cause many types of diseases, and is often associated with black magic and various minority groups in China.

When the patient eats meat, this stops. Sometimes when the snake *gǔ* leaps up to the heart, the heart becomes distended and the patient wants to vomit. Also, this thing in the body is sometimes there and sometimes not there for up to four or five years but then it takes on form and can bite. There are also those that mutate into a fleshy turtle or tortoise in order to bite. The snake moves and bites in the skin and the belly until it is old; some days it bites twenty or thirty times. At this time when the internal snake turns around to bite, the patient comes down with fever, scorched-looking forehead, and headache, as if he were being stung by ants. At night is is more severe. This is the external snake of a *gǔ* household, arriving from the wind. Internal snakes bite the organs; external snakes enter through the pores. This snake is formless. It is also countless in number.

用雄黃（五錢，研末）、生菖蒲（四兩）、蒜子（四兩）。搗爛，三味缺一不可，同放浴盆內，倒熱水於內，令病者自頭至腳，處處洗到，隔日一洗，以禦外蛇。

Use: *xióng huáng* (five *qián*, ground into a powder), *shēng chāng pú* (four *liǎng*), *suàn zǐ* (four *liǎng*). Pound the above into a pulp. You cannot omit even one of these three medicinals. Place them all together in a bath tub and pour in hot water. Make the patient wash everywhere from head to foot. Wash like this every other day. This is used to defend against external snakes.

再用馬兜鈴（四兩）同水久煨，多服。服藥後，忌食茶水飲食半日。若蛇不能吐出瀉下，仍將蘇荷湯四方（見後）加減治。服過半月，復用馬兜鈴半斤煎濃湯服。如此三五次，其蛇自化不見。愈後仍戒雞鴨二年，魚蝦螺蚌等戒三年，終身戒食蛇蛤。

Then use *mǎ dōu líng* (four *liǎng*) simmered in water for a long time. The patient should take a lot internally. After taking the medicine, avoid food, tea, or water; avoid drinking or eating for half a day. If the snakes cannot be vomited out or come out with diarrhea, treat with modifications of the four *Sū Hé Tāng*

(Perilla and Mint Decoction) formulas (see below).[113] After taking one of these formulas for half a month, have the patient take another half *jīn* of *mǎ dōu líng*, boiled into a concentrated decoction. After three or five times like this, the snake will automatically dissolve and disappear. After recovery, chicken and duck are still forbidden for two years. Fish, shrimp, snails, clams, and so forth are forbidden for three years. Snakes and frogs canot be eaten for the rest of the life.

有李姓妻者中此毒，內蛇長五六寸，日咬數十次，照方服藥，不戒鹽葷，兩月而愈。

There was a woman named Lǐ who was struck by these toxins. The internal snakes were five or six *cùn* long. Each day they bit her about ten times. She took one of these formulas and did not avoid salt and meat.[114] She recovered in two months.

陰蛇蠱 *Yīn Shé Gǔ*
Yīn Snake *Gǔ*

中此毒者，不出三十日多死。亦用雄黃末、蒜子、菖蒲搗爛，放熟水內。洗身以禦外蛇。若在酒內中毒，斷不可用酒罐煨藥，犯之必翻，愈翻則毒入愈深。茶內中毒，戒茶。病痊後可吃。

One who has been struck by this type of toxin often dies in less than thirty days. Again pound *xióng huáng* powder, *suàn zǐ* (garlic), and *chāng pú* into a pulp [as described in the previous entry]. Place them in hot water and bathe the body in order to defend against external snakes. If the poison was in liquor, you definitely cannot cook the medicine in a liquor jar. If you violate this, the patient

---

113. The four formulas are: 蘇荷湯 *Sū Hé Tāng* (Perilla and Mint Decoction), 槐芪湯 *Huái Qí Tāng* (Sophorae and Astragalus Decoction), 歸連湯 *Guī Lián Tāng* (Angelica and Forsythia Decoction), and 參芪湯 *Shēn Qí Tāng* (Glehnia and Astragalus Decoction). All of them contain *zǐ sū* and *bò hé*. The details of these formulas are given later in this chapter.

114. 葷 *hūn*, translated here as meat, can also mean the strong-smelling vegetables, such as garlic, onions, leek, etc. This term is used a number of times in this chapter.

will relapse. The more he relapses, the deeper the toxins penetrate. If the poison was in tea, tea is forbidden. These can be eaten again after the disease recovers.

無力者常煎紫蘇、薄荷二味作茶吃。有力者照後蘇荷湯四方加減治服。

Someone who is weak should often drink a tea made by boiling *zǐ sū* and *bò hé*. Someone who is strong should be treated by taking the modified the four *Sū Hé Tāng* (Perilla and Mint Decoction) formulas.

癲蠱 *Diān Gǔ*
Madness *Gǔ*

獞俗埋蛇土中，取毒菌，食則人心昏頭眩，笑罵無常；或遇飲酒時，藥毒輒發，忿怒兇狠；不可制者，名曰癲蠱。照薄荷煎四方治之，必須戒色。

A custom of the Zhuàng 獞 ethnic group [of Guǎngxī] is to bury snakes in the earth [to grow] a poisonous mushroom. When eaten, the victim's heart-mind becomes cloudy and his head dizzy. He alternates between laughing and scolding. Or if he happens to drink liquor, toxins from the drug come out, leading to fury and violence. When this is uncontrollable, it is called madness *gǔ*. Treat it according to the four *Sū Hé Jiān* formulas [see below in this chapter]. He must abstain from sex.

腫蠱 *Zhǒng Gǔ*
Swelling *Gǔ*

受毒者，肚必常叫。獞俗謂之放腫，腹大而鳴，大便結秘；甚則一耳常塞，一耳少厚。方用蘇荷湯四方。若病危甚時，必戒鹽葷方效。外用茨菇菜煎水洗之。

The belly of someone who has received these toxins will constantly call out. The Zhuàng ethnic group commonly calls this letting out swelling. The abdomen becomes enlarged and gurgles. The stool becomes bound up. When it is severe, one ear is constantly blocked and the other ear becomes a little swollen. Use the four *Sū Hé Tāng* (Perilla and Mint Decoction) formulas. When the disease is critical and severe, he must avoid salt and meat for this to be effective. Externally, wash him with water in which *cí gū cài* was boiled.

疳蠱 *Gān Gǔ*
Gān[115] *Gǔ*

宜用槐連湯：連翹（ 五錢 ）、條參（ 五錢 ）、青蒿（ 一兩 ）、生地（ 五錢 ）、槐花（ 一兩 ）、元參（ 五錢 ）、黃連（ 二錢 ）、貝母（ 五錢 ）、黃芩（ 五錢 ）。

You should use *Huái Lián Tāng*:

lián qiáo	連翹	5 *qián*
tiáo shēn	條參	5 *qián*
qīng hāo	青蒿	1 *liǎng*
shēng dì	生地	5 *qián*
huái huā	槐花	1 *liǎng*
yuán shēn	元參	5 *qián*
huáng lián	黃連	2 *qián*
bèi mǔ	貝母	5 *qián*
huáng qín	黃芩	5 *qián*

右水煎服 。

Boil the above in water and have the patient take it internally.

---

115. 疳 *gān* refers to 1) A childhood disease with emaciation and abdominal distention often attributed to worms, or 2) Various kinds of ulcerations and sores that eat away the flesh.

中害神 *Zhòng Hài Shén*
Harm-Striking Spirit

放害神 。亦蠱類也 。人中其藥則額必焦，口腥 、神昏 、性躁 、目見邪鬼形 、耳聞邪鬼聲，如犯大罪，如有刀兵健卒追趕，常思自盡 。治方，用柴胡湯加減服，宜戒鹽葷，俟毒淨自愈 。愈後，不用戒魚蝦等物 。

The harm-releasing spirit is also a type of *gǔ*. When someone is struck by this drug, his forehead looks burnt, his mouth smells fishy, his spirit is clouded, his temperament is agitated, his eyes see evil ghost shapes, and his ears hear evil ghost sounds. He acts as if he has committed a felony, as if there were armed soldiers pursuing him, and he constantly thinks of suicide. The formula to treat this is modified *Chái Hú Tāng*. He will automatically recover if he avoids salt and meat, and waits for the toxins to be cleaned out. After recovery, he does not need to avoid things like fish and shrimp.

柴胡湯：生地（ 四錢 ）、白芍 、知母 、元參 、生芪 、連翹（ 各三錢 ）、柴胡（ 一兩 ）、百合（ 五錢 ）、青蒿（ 六錢 ）、天冬（ 一錢 ）。

Chái Hú Tāng:

shēng dì	生地	4 *qián*
bái sháo	白芍	3 *qián*
zhī mǔ	知母	3 *qián*
yuán shēn	元參	3 *qián*
shēng qí	生芪	3 *qián*
lián qiáo	連翹	3 *qián*
chái hú	柴胡	1 *liǎng*
bǎi hé	百合	5 *qián*
qīng hāo	青蒿	6 *qián*
tiān dōng	天冬	1 *qián*

水煎服。

Boil the above in water and have the patient take it internally.

又方：夏枯草（二兩）、紫背浮萍（三錢），右水煎服。

Another formula: Boil *xià kū cǎo* (two *liǎng*) and *zǐ bèi fú píng* (two *qián*) in water and have the patient take it internally.

金蠶蠱 *Jīn Cán Gǔ*
Golden Silkworm *Gǔ*

此蠱金色，其形如蠶，能入人腹，食人腸胃、其糞亦能毒人。養蠱之家，蓄以害人，用金銀等物將蠱送之路旁，有人遇之，蠱即隨往，謂之嫁金蠶。此蠱不畏水火刀槍，最難滅除。惟畏刺。中此蠱者食白礬味甜，嚼黑豆不腥者即是。又初吃藥後，周身皮肉如有數百蟲行，癢極難忍者亦是。用石榴皮根煎湯飲之，可以吐出。

This *gǔ* is golden-colored and is shaped like a silkworm. It can enter a person's abdomen, eating his intestines and stomach and its excrement can also poison the person. Households that raise *gǔ* and save it to harm people use gold and silver things to carry the *gǔ* to the roadside. When they encounter someone, they give him the *gǔ* and follow along, calling it marriage of the golden silkworm. This *gǔ* does not fear water, fire, swords, or spears and is most difficult to eliminate. When someone who is struck by this *gǔ* eats *bái fán*, it tastes sweet, and when he chews black soybeans, they do not taste fishy. Also, after initially taking herbs, the skin and flesh of the entire body feels like it has several hundred insects crawling on it, with extreme itching that is difficult to endure. Induce vomiting by drinking a decoction of *shí liú pí gēn*.

又方：常山（四錢）、山荳根（五錢）、蜈蚣（一條烘乾）、黃柏（五錢）、蜘蛛（五隻，烘乾）、穿山甲（五錢）、白鴿血（一隻全血，烘乾）。

Another formula:

cháng shān	常山		4 *qián*
shān dòu gēn	山豆根		5 *qián*
wú gōng	蜈蚣	dried over a fire	1 *pc*
huáng bǎi	黃柏		5 *qián*
zhī zhū	蜘蛛	dried over a fire	5 spiders
chuān shān jiǎ	穿山甲		5 *qián*
bái gē xuè	白鴿血	dried over a fire	all the blood of one pigeon

以上七味，同研末，分三次，泡滾酒服，其毒自化。毒重者
服此方必愈。不用戒口。

Powder the above seven herbs together, and divide it into three doses. Steep it in boiling liquor and have the patient take it. The toxins will automatically dissolve. If the toxins are serious, the patient will recover after taking this formula. There is no need for a special diet.

中疳中蛇中腫中癲諸方
Zhōng Gān Zhōng Shé Zhōng Zhǒng Zhōng Diān Zhū Fāng
Various Formulas for *Gān* Strike, Snake Strike, Swelling Strike, and Madness Strike

蘇荷湯：紫蘇[116]、南薄荷、青蒿（各一兩）、條參、連翹
（各八錢）、槐花、元參（各七錢）、柴胡（六錢）、川芎
（二錢）、生芪（五錢）。

Sū Hé Tāng (Perilla and Mint Decoction):

zǐ sū	紫蘇	1 *liǎng*
nán bò hé	南薄荷	1 *liǎng*
qīng hāo	青蒿	1 *liǎng*
tiáo shēn	條參	8 *qián*

116. In this and the following formulas, 紫蘇 *zǐ sū* may refer to 紫蘇葉 *zǐ sū yè*, or to all the above-ground parts of the plant.

lián qiáo	連翹	8 *qián*
huái huā	槐花	7 *qián*
yuán shēn	元參	7 *qián*
chái hú	柴胡	6 *qián*
chuān xiōng	川芎	2 *qián*
shēng qí	生芪	5 *qián*

按：蛇蠱加白芷（一兩）、三七（二錢）。

Note: For snake *gǔ*, add *bái zhǐ* (one *liǎng*) and *sān qī* (two *qián*).

右受毒重者，水煎服。服藥之後病漸減者，即是對症，久服
自愈。大便秘結者，加茨菇菜一兩，更妙。

For a serious case of poisoning, boil the above in water and have the patient
take it. If the disease gradually improves after taking the medicine, the formula
is in accordance with the pattern. If the patient takes it for a long time, he will
automatically recover. If the patient has constipation, adding one *liǎng* of *cí gū
cài* is even more wonderful.

上方條參清肺火，消腫脹，連翹瀉心火，敗毒，紫蘇入肺、
心、脾，殺蛇發表，薄荷入肺殺蠱，槐花清肝火解毒，生黃
敗毒發表，元參清腎火解毒，川芎發表、青蒿殺蠱解毒。

In the above formula, *tiáo shēn* clears fire from the lungs, disperses swelling
and distention; *lián qiáo* drains heart fire and vanquishes toxins; *zǐ sū* enters
the lungs, heart, and spleen, kills snakes, and effuses the exterior; *bò hé* enters
the lungs and kills *gǔ*; *huái huā* clears liver fire and resolves toxins, *shēng huáng
qí* vanquishes toxins and effuses the exterior; *yuán shēn* clears kidney fire and
resolves toxins; *chuān xiōng* resolves toxins; and *qīng hāo* kills *gǔ* and resolves
toxins.

凡中蠱治方，大要不外殺蛇解毒，發毒敗毒之品。

Generally for formulas to treat *gǔ* strike, the main idea is nothing beyond materials to kill snakes, resolve toxins, send the toxins out, and vanquish the toxins.

槐芪湯：凡口乾火盛者，此方主之。槐花、青蒿（各一兩）、生地、紫蘇、南薄荷、連翹（各七錢）、生黃芪、天冬、元參、花粉（各五錢）、黃柏（三錢）。

Huái Qí Tāng (Sophorae and Astragalus Decoction): This formula is indicated whenever there is dry mouth with fire exuberance.

huái huā	槐花	1 *liǎng*
qīng hāo	青蒿	1 *liǎng*
shēng dì	生地	7 *qián*
zǐ sū	紫蘇	7 *qián*
nán bò hé	南薄荷	7 *qián*
lián qiáo	連翹	7 *qián*
shēng huáng qí	生黃芪	5 *qián*
tiān dōng	天冬	5 *qián*
yuán shēn	元參	5 *qián*
huā fěn	花粉	5 *qián*
huáng bǎi	黃柏	3 *qián*

頭痛加白芷（三錢）、川芎（二錢）。水煎服。

For headache add *bái zhǐ* (three *qián*) and *chuān xiōng* (two *qián*). Boil the above in water and have the patient take it internally.

歸連湯：當歸、生白芍（各三錢）、生地、連翹、百合、紫蘇、蘇薄荷（各五錢）、川芎、槐花、黃連、生甘草（各二錢）。

Guī Lián Tāng (Angelica and Forsythia Decoction):

dāng guī	當歸	3 *qián*
shēng bái sháo	生白芍	3 *qián*
shēng dì	生地	5 *qián*
lián qiáo	連翹	5 *qián*
bǎi hé	百合	5 *qián*
zǐ sū	紫蘇	5 *qián*

sū bò hé	蘇薄荷	5 *qián*
chuān xiōng	川芎	2 *qián*
huái huā	槐花	2 *qián*
huáng lián	黃連	2 *qián*
shēng gān cǎo	生甘草	2 *qián*

水煎服。腹脹除甘草。大便結秘，加茨菇菜一兩。

Boil the above in water and have the patient take it internally. If there is abdominal distention, remove *gān cǎo*. If there is constipation, add *cí gū cài* (one *liǎng*).

參芪湯：條參（ 七錢 ）、生黃芪、紫蘇、南薄荷、麥冬（ 去心 ）、青蒿（ 各五錢 ）、川芎（ 四錢 ）、茯苓（ 三錢 ）、百合、生地（ 各二錢 ）、連翹（ 一錢 ）。

Shēn Qí Tāng (Glehnia and Astragalus Decoction):

tiáo shēn	條參		5 *qián*
shēng huáng qí	生黃芪		5 *qián*
zǐ sū	紫蘇		5 *qián*
nán bò hé	南薄荷		5 *qián*
mài dōng	麥冬	remove the core	5 *qián*
qīng hāo	青蒿		5 *qián*
chuān xiōng	川芎		4 *qián*
fú líng	茯苓		3 *qián*
bǎi hé	百合		2 *qián*
shēng dì	生地		2 *qián*
lián qiáo	連翹		1 *qián*

右水煎服。

Boil the above in water and have the patient take it internally.

153

以上四方，皆治蠱要藥，治疳蠱更效。受毒者隨時加減服。藥不外四方內藥品。受毒極重者，戒鹽葷女色，服藥數月後，開葷鹽近色無妨，仍舊照方服藥一年，或二、三年。

These four formulas are all important medicines for treating *gǔ*, and are even more effective for treating *gān gǔ*. At all times after someone has received these toxins, modify and give him these formulas. No medicine is needed beyond these four formulas. If the patient has received an extremely serious case of toxins, he must avoid salt, meat, and female charms, as well as take the medicine for several months. Once he returns to a diet with meat and salt, and approaches women again without ill effects, he must still take the medicine for a year, or two or three years.

蘇荷生地湯：紫蘇、南薄荷、青蒿（各一兩）、生地、條參、連翹（各八錢）、槐花（七錢）、柴胡（六錢）、川芎（二錢）、生黃芪（五錢）。

Sū Hé Shēng Dì Tāng (Perilla, Mint, and Rehmannia Decoction):

zǐ sū	紫蘇	1 *liǎng*
nán bò hé	南薄荷	1 *liǎng*
qīng hāo	青蒿	1 *liǎng*
shēng dì	生地	8 *qián*
tiáo shēn	條參	8 *qián*
lián qiáo	連翹	8 *qián*
huái huā	槐花	7 *qián*
chái hú	柴胡	6 *qián*
chuān xiōng	川芎	2 *qián*
shēng huáng qí	生黃芪	5 *qián*

煎服。與前四方同功。大便結秘者，重加槐花、黃柏、黃芩、茨菇菜等味。小便赤者，加元參、梔子、茯苓。

Boil the above and have the patient take it internally. This gives the same results as the four formulas mentioned above. If there is constipation, double the *huái huā* and add medicinals such as *huáng bǎi*, *huáng qín*, and *cí gū cài*. If urine is red, add *yuán shēn*, *zhī zǐ*, and *fú líng*.

154

肝火盛者，加生白芍。頭痛加白芷。蛇蠱加白芷一兩、三七二錢。或帶熱嗽或咳血者，紫蘇、薄荷減半，加百合、麥冬、生芍各一兩。或時而傷風帶寒嗽者，去條參、連翹、槐花、青蒿、生地，加乾薑、當歸、半夏、陳皮、白芷。或人弱帶痢者，去條參、連翹、槐花、柴胡、生芪、青蒿、生地，加百合、白芍、茯苓、麥冬、砂仁、白朮、乾薑。

- For someone with effulgent liver fire, add *shēng bái sháo*.
- For headache add *bái zhǐ*.
- For snake *gǔ*, add *bái zhǐ* (one *liǎng*) and *sān qī* (two *qián*).
- For hot cough or coughing blood, halve the *zǐ sū* and *bò hé*; add *bǎi hé*, *mài dōng*, and *shēng [bái] sháo* (one *liǎng* of each).
- If from time to time wind damage carries cold cough with it, remove *tiáo shēn*, *lián qiáo*, *huái huā*, *qīng hāo*, and *shēng dì*; and add *gān jiāng*, *dāng guī*, *bàn xià*, *chén pí*, and *bái zhǐ*.
- If a weak person suffers dysentery, remove *tiáo shēn*, *lián qiáo*, *huái huā*, *chái hú*, *shēng qí*, *qīng hāo*, and *shēng dì*; and add *bǎi hé*, *bái sháo*, *fú líng*, *mài dōng*, *shā rén*, *bái zhú*, and *gān jiāng*.

總之，神而明之，存乎其人。但蠱毒未淨，不可服補藥與收斂藥。或兼有別病，則兼治之，而紫蘇、薄荷則斷不可去也。

In short, the patient's spirit will brighten up and will be retained within the person. But if the *gǔ* toxins are not cleaned out yet, he cannot take supplementing or astringing medicinals. When someone has a different disease at the same time, treat it at the same time, but you absolutely cannot remove the *zǐ sū* and *bò hé*.

又口舌熱爛，實火炎上，則去紫蘇、薄荷，重加槐花、黃柏、黃芩、茯苓、白芍、元參、澤瀉、天冬、石膏等味，酒水煨服。

Also, if the mouth and tongue are hot and putrid, repletion fire is flaring upward: remove the *zǐ sū* and *bò hé*; double the *huái huā*; and add *huáng bǎi*, *huáng qín*, *fú líng*, *bái sháo*, *yuán shēn*, *zé xiè*, *tiān dōng*, and *shí gāo*. Take it after decocting in liquor and water.

老人中蛇蠱方 *Lǎo Rén Zhōng Shé Gǔ Fāng*
Formula for an Elderly Person Stuck by Snake *Gǔ*

百合（四錢）、蘇子、南薄荷、當歸、茯苓、白芷、白芍
（各三錢）、麥冬、連翹（各二錢）。

bǎi hé	百合	4 *qián*
sū zǐ	蘇子	3 *qián*
nán bò hé	南薄荷	3 *qián*
dāng guī	當歸	3 *qián*
fú líng	茯苓	3 *qián*
bái zhǐ	白芷	3 *qián*
bái sháo	白芍	3 *qián*
mài dōng	麥冬	2 *qián*
lián qiáo	連翹	2 *qián*

水煎服。

Boil in water and have the patient take it internally.

又方：南薄荷、蘇子、麥冬、白芷、當歸（各三錢）、三
七、生首烏（各二錢）、連翹（四錢）、廣陳皮、木香
（各五分）、百合（五錢）。

Another formula:

nán bò hé	南薄荷	3 *qián*
sū zǐ	蘇子	3 *qián*
mài dōng	麥冬	3 *qián*
bái zhǐ	白芷	3 *qián*
dāng guī	當歸	3 *qián*
sān qī	三七	2 *qián*
shēng shǒu wū	生首烏	2 *qián*
lián qiáo	連翹	4 *qián*
guǎng chén pí	廣陳皮	5 *fēn*

mù xiāng	木香	5 *fēn*
bǎi hé	百合	5 *qián*

水煎服。

Boil the above in water and have the patient take it internally.

通治蠱方 *Tōng Zhì Gǔ Fāng*
Universal Formulas for Treating *Gǔ*

毒在上者，用升麻煎湯吐之，在腹者用鬱金煎湯下之，或合
二味服之，不吐則瀉，活人甚捷。

If the *gǔ* toxins are in the upper body, boil *shēng má* into a decoction to vomit
them out. If they are located in the abdomen, boil *yù jīn* to send them down
with the stool. Or combine the two herbs and take them; if the toxins aren't
vomited out, they will come out with the stool. This is an extremely quick way
to return the person to life.

又方：一覺腹中不快，即以生黃豆食之，入口不聞腥氣者，
此中蠱也，急以升麻濃煎湯飲，以手摳吐即愈，極效。如食
豆而腥者，即非蠱也。

Another formula: If someone perceives discomfort in the abdomen, he should
eat some fresh soybeans. If they don't smell fishy as they enter his mouth, he has
been struck by *gǔ*. He will recover when he quickly drinks a thick decoction of
shēng má and uses his hand to induce vomiting. This is extremely effective. If
he eats the beans but there is no fishy odor, it is not *gǔ*.

又方：先取炙甘草一寸，嚼之咽汁，若中蠱毒，隨即吐出，
仍以炙甘草三兩，生薑四兩，水煎，日三服。若含甘草而不
吐者，則非蠱毒。此蓋蠱家秘傳也。

Another formula: First chew a one-*cùn* long piece of *zhì gān cǎo*, swallowing
the juice. If struck by *gǔ* toxins, the patient will then vomit the juice back out.
Then boil three *liǎng* of *zhì gān cǎo* and four *liǎng* of fresh ginger in water. And

give three doses per day. If the patient holds the *gān cǎo* in his mouth without vomiting, then it is not *gǔ* toxins. This must have been handed down for generations in *gǔ* households.

又方：五倍子（ 二兩 ）、硫黃末（ 一錢 ）、甘草（ 三寸一半 微炒一半生用 ）、丁香、木香、麝香（ 各一分 ）、輕粉 （ 三分 ）、糯米（ 二十粒 ）。

Another formula:

wǔ bèi zǐ	五倍子		2 *liǎng*
liú huáng	硫黃	powder	1 *qián*
gān cǎo	甘草	three *cùn*, lightly stir-fried half of it, use half fresh	1 *fēn*
dīng xiāng	丁香		1 *fēn*
mù xiāng	木香		1 *fēn*
shè xiāng	麝香		1 *fēn*
qīng fěn	輕粉		3 *fēn*
nuò mǐ	糯米	glutinous rice	20 grains

入小砂罐內煎服 。（ 木香忌火，磨水兌服 。 ）服後，用高枕 平正仰臥，腹中如有物衝心，不必驚動，預備瓦缽，以便嘔 吐 。吐出惡物，吐罷飲茶一杯，瀉亦無妨。少時服食白粥。 忌生冷油膩酢醬。十日後，再服解毒丸兩三粒，即愈 。

Put the above into a small coarse clay container,[117] boil it and have the patient take it internally. (*Mù xiāng* should avoid fire; grind it, add to the water, and have the patient take it). After taking the formula, use a fat pillow and have the patient lie face up, flat and straight. He will feel as if there is something in his abdomen rushing into his heart. You must not be alarmed; be prepared with an earthenware bowl for vomiting as he will vomit out malign substances. When the vomiting stops, he should drink a cup of tea. There is also no harm if diarrhea occurs. After a short while, have him eat plain rice congee. He should avoid fresh, cold, oily, or greasy foods, vinegar, and sauces. After ten days, the

---

117. 砂罐 *shā guàn* (coarse clay container): 砂 *shā* refers to sand, sandstone, or perhaps some kind of coarse clay. Since it is used for decoction, it is more likely to mean coarse clay than sandstone.

patient should then take two or three *Jiě Dú Wán* (Resolve Toxins Pills).[118] He will then recover.

辟蠱毒法 *Pì Gǔ Dú Fǎ*
Methods of Repelling *Gǔ* Toxins

將食時，自帶生大蒜頭食之，有蠱必當場吐出，不吐則死，主人畏累，則不敢下蠱。

At the time of eating a meal, a person should carry his own head of fresh garlic and eat it. If there is *gǔ*, right then and there they will be vomited out. If not vomited out, they will die. When the host fears trouble, he will not dare to put *gǔ* in the food.

又方：大荸薺，不拘多少，切片，晒乾，為末，每早空心白滾湯調下二錢，入蠱家無害，此神方也。

Another formula: Slice an unlimited quantity of big water chestnuts, dry them in the sun, and powder them. Each morning on an empty stomach take two *qián* in plain boiled water. There will be no harm when entering a *gǔ* household; this is a miraculous formula.

又方：凡不飲酒之人，受蠱輕而易治，飲酒者受蠱重而難治。蠱毒多在煙瘴邊地，凡有煙瘴之處，又宜飲酒以辟瘴氣。是亦不能不飲，總之，在家多飲，出外少飲為妙。

Another formula: Whenever someone who does not drink liquor receives *gǔ*, it will be light and easy to treat, but someone who drinks and receives *gǔ* will have a more serious case that is difficult to treat. *Gǔ* toxins are often found in a miasmic border districts, but whenever places are miasmic, it is also appropriate to drink liquor in order to repel miasmic qì. One must still drink, so in short, when at home drink a lot, but it is wonderful to drink less while traveling.

---

118. 解毒丸 *Jiě Dú Wán* (Resolve Toxins Pills): There is no formula with this name in《驗方新編》*Yàn Fāng Xīn Biān*. It may refer to a formula by that name in Volume 10 of the《三因極一病證方論》*Sān Yīn Jí Yī Bìng Zhèng Fāng Lùn* by 陳言 Chén Yán (宋) *Sòng* Dynasty. See appendix on p. 201.

Chapter 11

瘴癘 *Zhàng Jī*
Miasma and Pestilence

Translator's Note: This chapter takes a few recipes from Volume 15 of 《驗方新編》 *Yàn Fāng Xīn Biān*.

解煙瘴毒 *Jiě Yān Zhàng Dú*
Resolving Miasmic Toxins

用瓷瓦有鋒者，或刺額上 、或刺眉叢 、或刺兩手膊 、出血一升即解 。血紅而多者輕，血紫而少者重 。

Let blood by pricking with the sharp edge of a porcelain tile: above the forehead or the clump of the eyebrows or both hands and arms. The condition will resolve after one *shēng* of blood has been let out. In a light case, the blood is red and copious; in a severe case, it is purple and scant.

又方：白朮 、陳皮 、茯苓 、半夏 、栀仁 、山查 、神麯（ 各一錢 ）、連翹 、前胡 、蒼朮（ 各七分 ）、生甘草（ 四分 ）。

It is appropriate to use:

bái zhú	白朮	1 *qián*
chén pí	陳皮	1 *qián*
fú líng	茯苓	1 *qián*
bàn xià	半夏	1 *qián*
zhī rén	栀仁	1 *qián*
shān zhá	山查	1 *qián*

160

shén qū	神麯	1 *qián*
lián qiáo	連翹	7 *fēn*
qián hú	前胡	7 *fēn*
cāng zhú	蒼术	7 *fēn*
shēng gān cǎo	生甘草	4 *fēn*

右生薑引，煎服數劑，神效。凡客遊不服水土者。亦效。

The above are conducted by *shēng jiāng*.[119] Boil it and give the patient several doses. It has miraculous effects. This is also effective whenever a traveler has not acclimatized.

又方：生、熟大蒜各七片，共食之，少頃腹鳴，或吐血或大便，即愈。

Another formula: Eat seven slices each of fresh and cooked garlic. In a short while, there will be abdominal gurgling, or vomiting blood, or a bowel movement, and then recovery.

避煙瘴癘 Bì Yān Zhàng Jī
Averting Miasma and Pestilence

凡雲、貴、兩廣等省地方，忽有一股香味撲鼻，即是瘴氣。斷不可聞，以免生病。

Whenever you are in regions such as Yúnnán, Guìzhōu, Guǎngdōng, and Guǎngxī provinces, your nose may suddenly be assailed by an exotic odor. This is miasmic qì. Absolutely do not smell it if you want to avoid falling ill.

又方：凡有瘴氣之處，飲食不可過飽。每日須飲酒數杯；不飲酒，亦勉飲強之，可避瘴氣。

Another formula: Whenever you are in a place with miasmic qì, you cannot eat and drink too much. You should drink several cups of liquor every day. You

---

119. In other words, add some ginger to the decoction. It will help take the formula where it needs to go.

must force yourself even if you do not drink liquor. This can avert miasmic qì.

有三人早行山霧中，一死、一病、一安然無恙。後乃知死者過於食飽，病者系空腹，無恙者飲酒也。

There were three people who went out into the mountain mists early one day. One died, one got sick, and one escaped unscathed. Afterwards, I realized that the one who died had overeaten, the one who got sick had gone out on an empty stomach, and the one who was unscathed had drunken liquor.

Chapter 12

瘟疫 *Wēn Yì*
Scourge Epidemics

Translator's Note: These recipes come from Volume 15 of 《 驗方新編 》 *Yàn Fāng Xīn Biān*.

瘟疫症 *Wēn Yì Zhèng*
Scourge Epidemic Diseases

此症多發於春分之後，夏至之前，故曰瘟疫。如有鬼癘之氣，又曰癘疫。以眾人所患相同，又曰天行時疫。其症與傷寒相似，傳經表裡，亦無不同。惟時令已暖，毒瓦斯郁蒸，與傷寒微異，發散宜用辛平等劑。

This disease often breaks out after the spring equinox and before the summer solstice, so it is called scourge epidemic.[120] If there is ghost pestilence qì, it is also called pestilence epidemic. When what is suffered by everybody is the same, it is also called heaven current seasonal epidemic. This disease resembles cold damage; it is transmitted through the channels from exterior to interior; this is still not different. But the season is already warm, and there is constrained and steaming toxicity, so it is a little different than cold damage. To disperse it, it is appropriate to use the acrid level class of formulas.

---

120. 瘟 *wēn* scourge is pronounced the same as 溫 *wēn* warm; in addition, the character looks similar. The weather between the spring equinox and the summer solstice is warm. The author is pointing out the linguistic connection.

瘟疫諸方 *Wēn Yì Zhū Fāng*
Various Formulas for Scourge Epidemics

白粳米三合，連鬚蔥頭十根，煮成稠粥，加好醋一酒鐘，再煮一二滾、食一碗，熱服取汗，自愈。已出汗者不用。

Boil into a thick porridge three *gě* of non-glutinous white rice and ten scallion-heads including the root whiskers. Add a small winecup of good quality vinegar and boil it again for one or two 'rollings.' For spontaneous recovery, induce sweating by eating a bowl while it is hot. If the patient is already sweating do not use this formula.

又方：松毛切碎，搗，每用二錢，酒沖服，日三服。

Another formula: Cut up pine needles and pound them. Each time, take two *qián* drenched in liquor, three doses per day.

又，刺少商穴即愈。

Another: Prick Shào Shāng (LU 11) for recovery.

辟瘟散 *Pì Wēn Sàn*
Repel Scourge Powder

製蒼朮（五錢）、桔梗、神麯（各三錢）、貫眾、滑石、熟大黃、明雄、厚朴（薑汁炒）、生甘草、法半夏、川芎、藿香（各二錢）、羌活、白芷、柴胡（炒）、防風、荊芥、細辛、前胡、枳殼（炒）、薄荷、陳皮（去白）、皂角（去筋子[121]）、硃砂、石菖蒲、公丁香、廣木香、草菓（煨用子[122]）、香薷（各一錢）。

zhì cāng zhú	製蒼朮	5 *qián*

---

121. *Zào jiǎo* is a long pod, resembling a string bean (long bean) in form. It seems to have a string or thread running the long way through it, which should be removed.

122. There are smaller seeds inside *cǎo guǒ*.

jié gěng	桔梗		3 *qián*
shén qū	神麯		3 *qián*
guàn zhòng	貫眾		2 *qián*
huá shí	滑石		2 *qián*
shú dà huáng	熟大黃		2 *qián*
míng xióng	明雄		2 *qián*
hòu pò	厚朴	stir-fried in ginger juice	2 *qián*
shēng gān cǎo	生甘草		2 *qián*
fǎ bàn xià	法半夏		2 *qián*
chuān xiōng	川芎		2 *qián*
huò xiāng	藿香		2 *qián*
qiāng huó	羌活		1 *qián*
bái zhǐ	白芷		1 *qián*
chái hú	柴胡	stir-fried	1 *qián*
fáng fēng	防風		1 *qián*
jīng jiè	荊芥		1 *qián*
xì xīn	細辛		1 *qián*
qián hú	前胡		1 *qián*
zhǐ qìao	枳殼	stir-fried	1 *qián*
bò hé	薄荷		1 *qián*
chén pí	陳皮	remove the white part	1 *qián*
zào jiǎo	皂角	remove the 'sinew' and seeds	1 *qián*
zhū shā	朱砂		1 *qián*
shí chāng pú	石菖蒲		1 *qián*
gōng dīng xiāng	公丁香		1 *qián*
guǎng mù xiāng	廣木香		1 *qián*
cǎo guǒ	草果	roasted, use the seeds	1 *qián*
xiāng rú	香薷		1 *qián*

右共研極細末，磁瓶收貯，勿令洩氣。每遇患者，先用二三分，吹入鼻內。再用三錢，滾薑湯沖服。體虛者，加台黨參（四錢），煎湯沖服。小兒每服一錢。凡病重者，三服即愈。

Grind the above together into an extremely fine powder, and store it in a porcelain bottle. Do not let qì leak [the bottle must be airtight]. Everytime you encounter a patient, first blow two or three *fēn* of the powder into his nose. Then decoct ginger, drench three *qián* of the powder with it, and have the patient take it. If his body is vacuous, add *tái dǎng shēn* (four *qián*), boil into a decoction, drench the powder with it and have the patient take it. The dose for children is one *qián* each time. Whenever the disease is serious, the patient will recover after three doses.

大頭瘟 *Dà Tóu Wēn*
Massive Head Scourge

此症頭面腫大，咽喉閉塞。急用延胡索錢半，皂角、川芎各一錢，藜蘆五分，躑躅花二分半，共為末，用紙捻蘸藥推入鼻中取嚏，日三五次，甚效。嚏出膿血者更妙。無嚏者難治。左右看病之人，用此取嚏，亦不傳染。

In this disease, the head and face swell up big and the throat is obstructed. Quickly powder together 1.5 *qián* of *yán hú suǒ*; one *qián* each of *zào jiǎo* and *chuān xiōng*; five *fēn* of *lí lú*; and 2.5 *fēn* of *zhí zhú huā*. Three or five times a day, roll up a piece of paper, dip it in the medicine, and push it into the patient's nose to make him sneeze. This is extremely effective. It is even more wonderful if he sneeze out pus and blood. If he doesn't sneeze, it is difficult to treat. When you see sick people on the left and right, use this to get a sneeze and the disease will not be transmitted.

又方：黑豆二合（炒焦），炙甘草一錢，水二鐘，煎八分，熱服，神效。

Another formula: Boil two *gě* of black soybeans (scorched-fried) and one *qián* of *zhì gān cǎo* in two cups of water. Boil it down to eighty percent and take it while it is hot. This is miraculously effective.

辟瘟諸方 *Pi Wēn Zhū Fāng*
Various Formulas to Repel Scourges

五更時投黑豆一大握於井中，勿使人見，凡飲水家俱無傳染。若食河水之處，各家於每日清晨投黑豆一撮於水缸內，全家無恙。

Throw a big handful of black soybeans into a well during the fifth watch (4 to 6 a.m.), but don't let anyone see you do it. The disease will not be transmitted to anyone in the family who drinks this water. If it is a place where the people use water from the river [not a well], each family should throw a scoop of black soybeans in their water vat every day in the early morning. The entire family will be safe and sound.

又方：雷丸、大黃（各四兩）、飛金箔（三十張）、硃砂（三錢水飛）、生明礬（一兩）。

Another formula:

léi wán	雷丸	4 *liǎng*
dà huáng	大黃	4 *liǎng*
fēi jīn bó	飛金箔	30 sheets
zhū shā	朱砂　water-grind	3 *qián*
shēng míng fán	生明礬	1 *liǎng*

右共研末，以水為丸，每服二錢。

Grind the above together into a powder. Make it into pills using water. Each dose is two *qián*.

又方：貫眾（一箇）、白礬（一塊）。右放水缸內，亦效。

Another formula: One piece of *guàn zhòng* and one lump of *bái fán*. Place the above inside a water jar. This is also effective.[123]

---

123. It seems this pot of water simply sits in the room and absorbs the scourge *qì*.

又方：向東桃枝煎湯，日浴二次，自然不染。

Another formula: Boil east-growing peach twigs into a decoction. Bathe in it twice a day. There will naturally be no transmission of the disease.

又方：蒼朮、雄黃、丹參、桔梗、白朮、川芎、白芷、藜蘆、菖蒲、皂角、川烏、甘草、薄荷（各五錢）、細辛、蕪夷（各三錢）。

Another formula:

cāng zhú	蒼朮	5 qián
xióng huáng	雄黃	5 qián
dān shēn	丹參	5 qián
jié gěng	桔梗	5 qián
bái zhú	白朮	5 qián
chuān xiōng	川芎	5 qián
bái zhǐ	白芷	5 qián
lí lú	藜蘆	5 qián
chāng pú	菖蒲	5 qián
zào jiǎo	皂角	5 qián
chuān wū	川烏	5 qián
gān cǎo	甘草	5 qián
bò hé	薄荷	5 qián
xì xīn	細辛	3 qián
wú yí	蕪夷	3 qián

右藥俱用生料，曬乾研末，燒薰。可辟瘟疫，屢試神驗。

Use all of the above medicinals as uncooked materials. Dry them in the sun and grind them into a powder. Heat them until fragrant. This can avert scourge epidemics. This has been repeatedly tested with miraculous experiences.[124]

---

124. This and the next two formulas are medicinal incense. The ingredients are heated to let off a fragrance or burned to release smoke which can avert disease. 燒 shāo can mean to heat or to burn. In China and Japan, there were many types of incense that were heated for their fragrance and others that were

又方：紅棗（二斤）、茵陳（八兩切碎）、大黃（八兩切片）。共燒煙薰，可免瘟氣。

Another formula: *hóng zǎo* (two *jīn*), *yīn chén* (eight *liǎng*, cut into pieces), *dà huáng* (eight *liǎng*, sliced). Heating the above together until smoking and fragrant can avert scourge qì.

又方：蒼朮（末）、紅棗。共搗為丸，如彈子大，時時燒之，可免時疫不染。

Another formula: Pound *cāng zhú* (powdered) and *hóng zǎo* together into pellets the size of a marble. Frequently heat them to avert seasonal epidemics.

---

burned for smoke.

Chapter 13

奇病 *Qí Bìng*
Unusual Diseases

Translator's Note: This chapter comes from Volume 16 of 《 驗方新編 》
Yàn Fāng Xīn Biān. As you will see, these are indeed unusual diseases!

頭頂生瘡五色，形如櫻桃；破則自頂分裂，連皮剝脫至足；
此症名肉人。常服牛乳自愈。

A five-colored sore that is shaped like a cherry erupts on the vertex of the head.
When it breaks, it splits from the vertex and the skin continuously peels off and
sheds down to the feet. This disease is called *meat person*.[125] The patient will
automatically recover if he constantly drinks cow's milk.

眉毛搖動，晝夜不眠，呼喚不應，飲食如常。用大蒜
（ 二兩 ）搗汁兌酒飲，自愈。

The eyebrows shake and move about, with inability to sleep day or night. The
patient shouts what he should not, but eats and drinks as usual. Crush garlic
(two *liǎng*) to extract the juice, add liquor, and have the patient drink it. He will
automatically recover.

頭面發熱，身有光色。用大蒜汁（ 五錢 ），酒調服。吐物如
蛇，即愈。

---

125. 肉人 *ròu rén*: This is called meat person because the skin peels off leaving the flesh or meat exposed over the whole body.

Feverish head and face with a shiny body. Mix the juice of garlic (five *qián*) with liquor and have the patient drink it. He will recover after vomiting something that looks like a snake.

面腫如斗，見人纔三寸長；此痰症也 。用瓜蒂（ 炒 ）、紅飯豆（ 各一錢 ）。右水煎服一二劑，使痰吐盡，腫消而愈 。再用黨參 、焦朮 、茯苓 、半夏（ 各三錢 ）、甘草（ 一錢 ）、陳皮（ 五分 ），右水煎服 。

The face swells as big as a *dòu*,[126] and he sees people as only three *cùn* tall. This is a phlegm pattern. Boil *guā dì* (stir-fried) and *hóng fàn dòu*[127] (one *qián* of each) in water and give the patient one or two doses. This makes him vomit out the phlegm completely. The swelling will disperse and the patient will recover. Then boil *dǎng shēn, jiāo zhú, fú líng, bàn xià* (three *qián* of each); *gān cǎo* (one *qián*), and *chén pí* (five *fēn*) in water and have the patient take it internally.

見一物如兩物；此好食魚鮮所致 。食薑 、醋加紫蘇水，數日即愈 。

Seeing one thing as if it were two things. This is caused by liking to eat seafood. The patient should eat ginger and vinegar, adding *zǐ sū* water. Recovery will come after several days.

見一物如兩物，或三四物；又見桌椅等物平正者，視之反歪斜；歪斜者，視之反平正；此胸膈有伏痰也 。用常山（ 五錢，酒煮 ）、黨參蘆（ 三錢 ）、甘草（ 一錢 ）、生薑（ 五片 ），右水二碗，煎八分，食遠服，吐痰而愈 。

Seeing one thing as if it were two, sometimes three or four things. Also seeing things that are level and straight, for example tables and chairs, as if they were crooked; seeing things are crooked as if they were level and straight. This is latent phlegm in the chest and diaphragm. Use *cháng shān* (five *qián*, boiled in liquor), *dǎng shēn lú* (three *qián*), *gān cǎo* (one *qián*), and *shēng jiāng* (five slices). Boil the above in two bowls of water down to eighty percent. The

---

126. A 斗 *dòu* is equivalent to ten *shēng*. It is sometimes translated as a peck, although this is not precise.

127. 紅飯豆 *hóng fàn dòu* is also known as 赤小豆 *chì xiǎo dòu*.

patient should take it between meals. Recovery will come after he vomits up the phlegm.

酒後嘔吐視物顛倒，治法見煙酒醉傷 。

Vomiting and seeing things upside down after drinking liquor. To treat this, see the above section on damage from smoking and alcohol intoxication.

眼花見諸般飛禽走獸，以手撲捉則無；此膽肝邪火也 。用棗仁、羌活、青葙子花（ 即草決明花 ）、元明粉（ 各一兩 ），右共為末，每服二兩，水一碗，煎七分，和渣飲之，一日三服即愈 。

Flowery [blurred] vision, seeing various types of birds and beasts, trying to catch them but nothing is there. This is evil fire of the gall bladder and liver. Powder *zǎo rén, qiāng huó, qīng xiāng zǐ huā*, and *yuán míng fěn* (one *liǎng* of each). The patient should take two *liǎng* each dose. Boil it in one bowl of water down to seventy percent. Drink it along with the dregs. Recovery comes after taking three doses in one day.

口鼻流出臭水，以碗盛之 ，內有魚蝦走動，捉之即化爲水；此肉壞也 。多食雞，自愈 。

Bad-smelling fluid is discharged from the mouth and nose. When you fill a bowl with it, there are fish and shrimp running about inside it. When you capture them, they melt into the water. This is the patient's flesh spoiling. The patient will automatically recover if he frequently eats chicken.

口鼻中氣常出不散，凝如黑蓋，過十日後，漸漸至肩胸，與肉相連，堅如鐵石 。澤瀉煎湯，飲三盞，連服五日，即安 。

An odor constantly comes out of the mouth and nose and doesn't disperse. It congeals like a black cover. After ten days, it gradually reaches the shoulders and chest, and merges with the flesh, as hard as iron or stone. Decoct *zé xiè* and have the patient drink three small-cups. He will be in good health after taking this continuously for five days.

172

身發寒熱，四肢堅硬如石；敲之作鐘磬聲。吳萸（二錢，先用熱水泡過），煎水；木香（二錢），右研末，兌服，自愈。

The patient has generalized aversion to cold and fever and his four limbs are as hard as stone; tapping on his body makes a sound like clock chimes. Boil *wú yú* (two *qián*, previously soaked in hot water) in water. Grind *mù xiāng* (two *qián*) into a powder. Add it [to the boiled *wú yú*] and have the patient take it. He will automatically recovery.

週身皮肉內滾滾如波浪聲，癢不可忍，抓之血出；此名氣奔症。用虎杖、台黨、青鹽（各二錢）、細辛（七分），右水煎，緩緩服。

There is rolling or surging within the skin and flesh of the entire body with wave-like sounds and unbearable itching that bleeds when scratched. This is called qì running pattern. Boil *hǔ zhàng, tái dǎng, qīng yán* (two *qián* of each) and *xì xīn* (seven *fēn*) in water. He should take it little by little.

皮膚中如有蟹行走，有聲如小兒啼哭；此筋肉化也。用雷丸、雄黃（各五錢），右共為末，摻豬肉片上，火中燒熟食之，即愈。

Feeling as if there were crabs walking about in the skin with sounds like a baby crying. This is a transformation in the sinews and flesh. Powder *léi wán* and *xióng huáng* (five *qián* of each) together and sprinkle it on a slice of pork. Roast it in a fire and eat it while it is hot. Recovery will follow.

皮膚間如蚯蚓鳴；此水濕生蟲也。用蚯蚓糞，敷患處一寸厚，鳴止。再用薏苡仁、茨實（各一兩）、白朮（五錢）、生甘草（三錢）、黃芩（二錢）、附子（三分）、防風（五分），右水煎服，即愈。此治濕則蟲無以養，又有生甘草以解毒殺蟲，防風去風而逐瘀，附子斬關而搗邪，所以奏功如神也。

Sounds resembling the gurgling of earthworms coming from between the skin.[128] This is due to 'bugs' engendered by water-damp. Apply *qiū yǐn fēn*

---

128. Apparently, earthworms can make a gurgling sound underground when

(earthworm excrement)[129] to the affected site, one *cùn* thick. The gurgling sound will stop. Then boil *yì yǐ rén*, *qiàn shí* (one *liǎng* of each); *bái zhú* (five *qián*), *shēng gān cǎo* (three *qián*), *huáng qín* (two *qián*), *fù zǐ* (three *fēn*), and *fáng fēng* (five *fēn*) in water and have the patient take it. Recovery will follow. When this treats dampness, the *chóng* have nothing to nourish them. The formula also has *shēng gān cǎo* which resolves toxins and kills 'bugs'; *fáng fēng* removes wind and expels stasis; *fù zǐ* breaks down the door and crushes the evils. As a result, this is as effective as a miracle.

周身發斑眼赤，鼻脹氣喘，毛髮硬如銅鐵；此胃中熱毒，結於下焦。用滑石、白礬（各一兩），右水二碗，煎至一碗，冷服即愈。（外用吳萸末，熱醋調敷兩腳心，週時一換，以愈為止，此法最妙。）

The entire body erupts in macules, with red eyes, nasal distention, panting, and the head and body hair is as hard as copper or iron. This is heat and toxins in the stomach, bound up in the lower burner. Place *huá shí* and *bái fán* (one *liǎng* of each) in two bowls of water and boil it down to one bowl. Let it cool and have the patient take it. Recovery will follow. (Externally apply *wú yú* powder mixed with hot vinegar to the hearts of both feet. Change it once a day, stopping upon recovery. This method is most wonderful.)

身上忽現蛇形，痛不可忍。外用雄黃末，豬油調搽。內用托裏解毒湯，即愈。氣旺者用荊防敗毒散，更妙。

Snake-shapes suddenly appear on the body with unendurable pain. Externally apply *xióng huáng* powder mixed with pork lard. Internally use *Tuō Lǐ Jiě Dú Tāng*.[130] Recovery will follow. If qì is effulgent, it is even more wonderful to use *Jīng Fáng Bài Dú Sǎn*.[131]

---

disturbed.

129. 蚯蚓糞 *qiū yǐn fèn* (earthworm excrement) probably means worm castings.

130. 托裏解毒湯 *Tuō Lǐ Jiě Dú Tāng* (Expel Pus and Resolve Toxins Decoction): Described in Volume 11 of 《驗方新編》 *Yàn Fāng Xīn Biān*. See appendix on p. 198.

131. 荊防敗毒散 *Jīng Fáng Bài Dú Sǎn* (Schizonepita and Saposhnikovia Toxin-Vanquishing Powder): Described in Volume 11 of《驗方新編》*Yàn Fāng Xīn Biān*. See appendix on p. 199.

又方：取雨滴磉石上苔痕，用水融化，噙之即消。

Another formula: Gather lichen that grows where rain drips on the plinth stone beneath a pillar or post, and dissolve it in water. When the patient holds it in his mouth, the condition will disperse.

遍身忽然肉出如錐，癢而且痛，不能飲食；此名血攤症。不速治，則潰爛膿出。急用赤皮葱燒灰淋洗。內服淡豆豉，湯數盞，自安。

Suddenly there are cone-shaped eruptions in the flesh all over the body, with itching, pain, and inability to drink or eat. This is called *vendor's stall blood pattern*.[132] If you do not treat it quickly, it ulcerates and pus comes out. Quickly reduce red-skinned scallion (*chì pí cōng*) to ash and drip-wash the body with it. Internally have the patient take several small-cups of decocted *dàn dòu chǐ*. This will automatically calm it.

遍身生燎泡，如甘棠梨；破則水流，其泡復生；內有小石一片，如指甲大；此症抽盡肌肉，難治。用三棱、莪朮（各一錢），右為末，酒調服，效。

Burn-blisters appearing like *gān táng lí*[133] erupt over the entire body. When the blisters break, fluid flows from them and then they erupt again. Inside them there is a small piece of stone the size of a fingernail. This pattern exhausts the muscles and flesh and is difficult to treat. Powder *sān léng* and *é zhú* (one *qián* of each), mix with liquor, and have the patient take it. It is effective.

自頭麻至心窩而死；或自足心麻至膝蓋而死。小孩糞（乾結者佳，稀者不用），陰乾瓦上燒枯，燒至煙盡為止。每服三錢豆腐漿調服。或用豆腐調服亦可，甚效。

Numbness travelling from the head down to the pit of the stomach, leading to death. Sometimes the numbness runs from the heart of the feet up to the kneecaps and leads to death. Child's excrement (*xiǎo hái fèn*, dry and formed

---

132. This is called *xuè tān zhèng* (vender's stall blood pattern) because the rash looks like a cluster of vender's stalls, with red pointed roofs.

133. 甘棠梨 *gān táng lí* (sweet birchleaf pear, Pyri Betulaefoliae Fructus) has round pea-sized fruits.

is good; do not use watery stool). Dry it on a tile in the shade until it is dehydrated, and then roast it until it finishes smoking. Each dose is three *qián* mixed with soy milk, taken internally. You can also mix it with tofu and have the patient take it. This is extremely wonderful.

又方：川楝子，燒灰為末，每服一錢，黃酒調下。（外用吳茱末，熱醋調敷兩腳心，一週時一換，以愈為止，此法最妙。）

Another formula: Reduce *chuān lián zǐ* to ashes and powder it. Each dose is one *qián* mixed with yellow liquor and swallowed down. (Externally apply *wú yú* powder mixed with hot vinegar to the hearts of both feet, and change it once a day. Stop upon recovery. This method is most wonderful.)

臨臥遍身虱出，血肉俱壞漸生漸多，舌尖出血，身齒俱黑，脣動鼻開。日飲鹽醋湯數碗；十日自愈。

Lice come out all over the entire body at bedtime. Blood and flesh both spoil, gradually growing, gradually increasing. The tip of the tongue bleeds, and the body and teeth both turn black. The lips tremble and the nostrils flare open. Every day drink several bowls of decocted salt and vinegar. The patient will automatially recover in ten days.

忽有人影，與己隨行，坐臥則成形，與己無異；此名離魂症。用黨參（五錢有力者用人參一錢，或用高麗參三錢亦可）、辰砂、茯苓（各三錢），右煎服數劑。候形影不見，再服十全大補湯。

Suddenly there is a human shadow accompanying the patient. It takes shape when sitting or lying down, just the same as the patient. This is called separating *hún* pattern. Use *dǎng shēn* (five *qián*, if the patient is strong, use one *qián* of *rén shēn*. Three *qián* of *gāo lí shēn* can also be used); *chén shā*, *fú líng* (three *qián* of each). Boil the above and have the patient take several doses. Wait until the shadow no longer appears; then have the patient take *Shí Quán Dà Bǔ Tāng*.[134]

---

134. 十全大補湯 *Shí Quán Dà Bǔ Tāng* (Perfect Major Supplementation Decoction): This formula comes from the《太平惠民和劑局方》*Tài Píng Huì Mín Hé Jì Jú Fāng* (Tàipíng Imperial Grace Pharmacy Formulas). See appendix on p. 199.

人前不食背地偷食，見人則避，面色黃瘦；此名鼠膈病，乃
食過夜鼠饞之涎所致。用十大功勞葉（一名鼠怕草，葉似蒲
扇，有五角，角有刺），焙乾為末，每早空心服一錢，酒
下，服至半月，即俞。

The patient will not eat in front of people but steals food behind their backs
and avoids people. His facial complexion is yellow and withered. This is called
mouse [or rat] diaphragm disease (鼠膈病 *shǔ gé bìng*). It is caused by eating
food contaminated by the saliva of a mouse that ate some of it during the night.
Use *shí dà gōng láo yè* (also named *shǔ pà cǎo*, Weed Feared by Mice. The
leaves are shaped like a rush-leaf fan. They have five points with thorns.) Stone-
bake until dry and powder it. The patient should take one *qián* each morning
on an empty stomach, swallowed down with liquor. He will recover after taking
it for a half a month.

臥牀四肢不能舉動，口說大話並喜說食物；此名失說物望病
也。病人如說食肉，便云與爾食豬肉一頓，病人聞之即喜，
以肉放病人前，臨要吃，卻不與吃；此乃失他物望也。不必
服藥；其人睡中口流涎出，自愈。

The patient lies in bed, unable to raise his four limbs, talking big talk and is fond
of speaking about food. This disease is called losing the thing he says he hopes
for. When the patient speaks of eating meat, he is happy to hear you say 'I'll eat
a meal of pork with you.' But the patient will not eat when you put the meat in
front of him. This is losing his hoped-for thing. He does not need to take medicine; he will automatically recover when he drools during sleep.

男婦病邪與邪物交，獨言獨笑，悲哭恍惚。雄明黃（研細）
、蒼朮（研細，各一兩）、松香（二兩），右先將松香燒
化，以虎爪和各藥末，為丸如彈子大，夜燒火籠中，令病人
坐其上，以被蒙住，露頭在外，扶住薰之，連薰三夜，邪物
自去。愈後，必然泄瀉。多服平胃散，自愈；內有蒼朮，最
能辟邪。終身忌食蟹蛤。

Male-female disease evils, and intercourse with evil things, talking to oneself,
laughing alone, sorrowful weeping and abstraction. *Xióng míng huáng* (finely
ground), *cāng zhú* (finely ground, one *liǎng* of each); *sōng xiāng* (two *liǎng*).
First reduce the *sōng xiāng* to ashes. Blend all the powdered medicinals with

177

hŭ zhǎo (tiger's claws). Make pills the size of marbles. At night heat the pills in a steaming basket. Make the patient sit over it. Cover him with a quilt, with his head outside. Support him and fume him. Fume him for three consecutive nights. The evil thing will automatically leave. After the patient has recovered, he will certainly have diarrhea. He will automatically recover when he takes a lot of *Píng Wèi Sàn*.[135] *Cāng zhú* is in it; this herb is most able to ward off evils.[136] For the rest of his life he must avoid eating crab or frog.

驅狐怪法：凡狐迷男女，白日用口吸精，夜間交媾如人。用桐油搽陰處，自去。或用珠蘭根搽之，則獸自死，即將獸肉曬乾為末服之，更妙。

Method for driving out fox demons: Whenever foxes bewilder males or females, they suck in essence with their mouths in broad daylight and appear as if they were human to have sexual intercourse at night. They will automatically leave if you rub *tóng yóu* into the yīn places [genital-anal region]. Or the beast will automatically die if you rub *zhū lán gēn* into this area. Then dry the beast's flesh in the sun, powder it and have the patient take it. This is even more wonderful.

灸鬼法：治一切邪祟癲狂，胡言亂語，踰牆上屋，尋死等症。以病人兩手大拇指，用線齊頭捆攏，用艾絨於兩指縫中，離指甲角一半分之處（名鬼哭穴），半在甲上，半在肉上，四處盡燒，一處不燒，其疾不愈。

Moxibustion method for ghosts: This treats all evil spirits, withdrawal and mania, nonsensical speech and raving, climbing up the walls of the house, attempting suicide, and such patterns. Bind both of the patient's thumbs together with string. Use mugwort floss on the crack between the two thumbs, on the site that is one half *fēn* from the corner of the nail (named the Ghost Crying Points). The moxa cone should be half on the nail and half on the flesh. These

---

135. 平胃散 *Píng Wèi Sàn* (Stomach-Calming Powder): This formula originally came from the《太平惠民和劑局方》*Tài Píng Huì Mín Hé Jì Jú Fāng*. See appendix on p. 200.

136. 蒼朮 *cāng zhú* has a reputation for repelling ghosts and other types of supernatural creatures, especially when burned or heated as medicinal incense, but even when used internally. For example, 李時珍 Lǐ Shízhēn discussed this in《本草綱目》*Běn Cǎo Gāng Mù*.

four places should all be burnt. If one of the four places[137] is not burnt, the patient will not recover.

鬼箭傷：身痛有青色 。用亂髮擦之；髮捲成團而硬者即是 。 用金銀花（ 一兩 ），煎水飲之，即愈 。

Wounds from ghost arrows: The body is painful and has black and blue [bruises]. Rub it with hair (Crinis Crinis).[138] This means hair rolled up into a hard ball. Boil one *liǎng* of *jīn yín huā* in water. He will recover after drinking it.

又方：山梔（ 炒 ）、灰麵（ 炒 ）、桃枝尖（ 七個 ）。右共搥 融，作餅貼之 。次日將餅取下，分作七丸，放炭火中燒之， 燒時聲響，即愈 。不愈，再燒，以愈為止 。

Another formula: *shān zhī* (stir-fried), *huī miàn*[139] (stir-fried), *táo zhī jiān* (peach twig tips, seven). Pound the above together until soft. Make it into cakes and apply them. The next day, remove the cakes. Divide them into seven pellets. Put them in a charcoal fire and burn them. They will make sounds while they are burning. The patient will then recover. If he doesn't recover, burn them again. Stop when he recovers.

又方：鐵渣（ 取細淨者，二兩 ）、核桃（ 又名胡桃，取淨 肉，一斤 ）、桃仁（ 八兩 ），右同入磁瓶內，加好酒四斤蒸 熟，每日不拘時，隨量飲酒，蓋被取汗 。服後，痛甚無妨， 越痛越好，服完自俞 。

Another formula: *tiě zhā* (iron dust, select fine clean pieces, two *liǎng*), *hé táo* (select clean flesh, one *jīn*), *táo rén* (eight *liǎng*). Put the above together inside a porcelain bottle, add four *jīn* of good liquor, and steam it. Each day, not sticking to any particular time, drink some of the liquor. Cover up with a quilt

---

137. These four places: 1) The nail of the right thumb; 2) the adjacent flesh of the right thumb; 3) the nail of the left thumb; and 4) the adjacent flesh of the left thumb.

138. 亂髮 *luàn fà*: According to Wiseman, this simply indicates hair. The term literally means 'chaotic hair.'

139. 灰麵 *huī miàn*, literally 'grey flour' is flour that is mixed with the juice of herbs, including 蓬柴草 *péng chái cáo*. This turns it grey, hence its name.

to promote sweating. After taking it, there is no harm if the pain is severe. More pain is better. He will automatically recover after taking all of it.

Herbs that are in grey are an alternate name or a processed form of the herb above them and have the same Botanical, Latin, and Common names.

Pinyin	Chinese	Botanical	Latin	Common
bā dòu	巴豆	*Fructus Crotonis*	*Croton tiglium*	Croton fruit
bái fán	白礬	*Alumen*	*Alunite*	Alum
bái fù zǐ	白附子	*Rhizoma Typhonii*	*Typhonium giganteum*	Giant Voodoo Lily
shēng bái fù zǐ	生白附子			Fresh
bái guǒ	白果	*Semen Ginkgo*	*Ginkgo blioba*	Gingko nuts
bái jí	白及	*Rhizoma Bletillae*	*Bletilla striata*	Common bletilla rubber
bái jiè zǐ	白芥子	*Semen Sinapis albae*	*Sinapis alba*	White mustard seed
bái méi	白梅	*Fructus Armeniacae Mume*	*Armeniaca mume*	Candied mume
bái mù ěr	白木耳	*Tremella*	*Tremella fuci formis*	Wood ear
bái sháo	白芍	*Radix Paeoniae alba*	*Paeonia lactiflora*	White peony root
chǎo bái sháo	炒白芍			stir-fried white paeony root
bái xiān pí	白鮮皮	*Cortex Dictamni*	*Dictamnus dasycarpus*	Densefruit pittany root-bark
bái zhǐ	白芷	*Radix Angelicae Dahuricae*	*Angelica dahurica*	Dahurian angelica root
bái zhú	白术	*Rhizoma Atractylodis Macrocephalae*	*Atractylodes macrocephala*	Largehead atractylodes rhizome
jiāo zhú	焦术			Parched
bǎi hé	百合	*Lilium lancifolium*	*Bulbus Lilii*	Lilly bulb
bàn xià	半夏	*Rhizoma Pinelliae*	*Pinellia ternata*	Pinellia tuber
fǎ bàn xià	法半夏			Processed pinellia tuber
fǎ xià	法夏			
shēng bàn xià	生半夏			Fresh pinellia tuber
zhì bàn xià	製半夏			Processed pinellia tuber
bèi mǔ	貝母	*Bulbus Fritillaria*	*Fritillaria*	Fritillaria
bí qí pí	荸薺皮	*Heleocharis tuberosa pericarpium*	*Heleocharis dulcis*	Water chestnut skin
bì má zǐ	蓖麻子		*Ricini semen*	Castor bean

184

biē jiǎ	鱉甲	Carapax Trionycis	Trionyx sinensis Wiegmann	Turtle carapace
bīng piàn	冰片	Borneolum	Borneolus	Borneol
bò hé	薄荷	Herba Menthae	Mentha haplocalyx, M.canadaensis, M. arvensis	Peppermint
nán bò hé	南薄荷			
cán dòu	蠶豆	Semen Viciae Fabae	Vicia faba Linn.	Broad beans (fava bean)
cán jiǎn	蠶繭	Incunabulum Bombycis	Bombyx mori	Silkworm cocoon
cāng ěr cǎo	蒼耳草	Herba Xanthium	Xanthium sibiricum Patrin.	Siberian cocklebur plant
cāng zhú	蒼朮	Rhizoma Atractylodis	Atractylodes lancea	Atractylodes rhizome
zhì cāng zhú	製蒼朮			Processed atractylodes rhizome
cǎo guǒ	草果	Fructus Tsaoko	Amomum tsaoko Crevost et Lemaire	Fruit of caoguo
chái hú	柴胡	Radix Bupleuri	Bupleurum chinense	Root of Chinese Thorowax
chāng pú	菖蒲	Rhizoma Acori Tatarinowii	Acorus tatarinowii Schott.	Grassleaf sweetflag rhizome
shēng chāng pú	生菖蒲			Fresh
shí chāng pú	石菖蒲			
cháng shān	常山	Radix Dichroae	Dichroa febrifuga Lour.	Antifebrile dichroa root
chén pí	陳皮	Pericarpium Citri Reticulatae	Citrus reticulata Blanco.	Dried tangerine peel
guǎng chén pí	廣陳皮			
chì pí cōng	赤皮葱			Red-skinned scallion
chuān bèi mǔ	川貝母	Bulbus Fritillariae Cirrhosae	Fritillaria cirrhosa	Tendril leaf fritillary bulb
chuān jiāo	川椒	Fructus Zanthoxylum	Zanthoxylum simulans	Sichuān pepper
chuān lián	川連	Rhizoma Coptidis	Coptis chinensis	Sichuān gold thread
chuān huáng lián	川黃連			
chuān shān jiǎ	穿山甲	Squama Manis	Manis pentadactyla Linnaeus	Pangolin scales
chuān wū	川烏	Radix Aconiti	Aconitum carmichaeli	Common monkshood mother root
chuān xiōng	川芎	Rhizoma Ligustici Chuanxiong	Ligusticum chuanxiong	Sichuan lovage rhizome

起
死
回
生

185

Pinyin	Chinese	Pharmaceutical	Botanical	English
chún jiǔ	醇酒			A good type of liquor
cí shí	磁石	*Magnetitum*		Magnetite
cì wèi pí	刺蝟皮	*Corium Erinacei Seu Hemiechini*	*Erinaceus europaeus* Linnaeus	Hedgehog pelt
dà huáng	大黃	*Radix et Rhizoma Rhei*	*Rheum palmatum*	Rhubarb root and rhizome
shú dà huáng	熟大黃			Wine cooked rhubarb root and rhizome
dà suàn	大蒜	*Bulbus Allii*	*Allium sativum*	Garlic
suàn zǐ	蒜子			
dàn dòu chǐ	淡豆豉	*Semen Sojae Preparatum*	*Glycine max*	Fermented soybean
dāng guī	當歸	*Radix Angelicae Sinensis*	*Angelica sinensis* (Oliv.) Diels, *A. polymorpha* Maxim	Chinese angelica
guī wěi	歸尾			Chinese angelica tail
dǎng shēn	黨參	*Radix Codonopsis*	*Codonopsis pilosula*	Codonopsis (Root of Pilose Asiabell)
tái dǎng shēn	台黨參			
dēng cǎo	燈草	*Medulla Junci*	*Juncus effusus*	Common rush
dēng xīn	燈心			
dì gǔ pí	地骨皮	*Cortex Lycii*	*Lycium chinense*	The root of *gǒu qǐ* 枸杞 (Chinese Wolfberry)
dì huáng	地黃	*Radix Rehmannia*	*Rehmannia glutinosa*	Foxglove root
dà shēng dì	大生地			
shēng dì	生地			Fresh
xiān dì huáng	鮮地黃			Fresh
dì yú	地榆	*Radix Sanguisorbae*	*Sanguisorba officinalis*	Garden burnet root
dīng xiāng	丁香	*Flos Caryophylli*	*Eugenia caryophyllata*	Clove
gōng dīng xiāng	公丁香			
dōng guā zhī	冬瓜汁	*Benincasa Recens*	*Benincasa hispida*	Fresh winter melon juice
dù zhòng	杜仲	*Cortex Eucommiae*	*Eucommia ulmoides* Oliver	Chinese rubber tree
chuān dù zhòng	川杜仲			Sìchuān Hardy rubber tree
é zhú	莪朮	*Rhizoma Curcumae*	*Curcuma aeruginosa*	Zedoary rhizome
fáng fēng	防風	*Radix Saposhnikoviae*	*Saposhnikovia divaricata*	Divaricate saposhnikovia root

Pinyin	Chinese	Pharmaceutical	Botanical	English
fáng jǐ	防己	*Radix Stephaniae Tetrandrae*	*Stephania tetrandra*	Mealy fangji [root]
fèng xiān huā gēn	鳳仙花根	*Radix Impatiens balsamina*	*Impatiens balsamina* (L.)	Garden Balsam, Rose Balsam
fù zǐ	附子	*Radix Aconiti Lateralis Preparata*	*Aconitum carmicheli* Debx.	Prepared common monkshood branched root
gān cǎo	甘草	*Radix et Rhizoma Glycyrrhizae*	*Glycyrrhiza uralensis* Fisch.	Licorice root
shēng gān cǎo	生甘草			Fresh
zhì cǎo	炙草			Honey-fried
gān yān zhī	乾胭脂		*Dactylopius coccus* Costa	Dried Cochineal
yān zhī chóng	胭脂蟲			
gǎn lǎn	橄欖	*Fructus Canarii Albi*	*Canarium album* (Lour.) Raeusch.	Chinese olive
gǎn lǎn hé	橄欖核	*Endocarpium et Semen Canarii*	*Canarium album* (Lour.) Raeusch.	Chinese olive pits
gāo lí shēn	高麗參	*Radix Ginseng Coreensis*	*Panax ginseng*	Korean ginseng
gǎo běn	藁本	*Rhizoma et Radix Ligustici*	*Ligusticum sinense* Oliv.	Root and rhizome of Chinese lovage
gé huā	葛花	*Flos Pueraria*	*Pueraria lobata* (Willd.) Ohwi	
gǔ suì bǔ	骨碎補	*Rhizoma Drynariae*	*Drynaria fortunei; D. roosii.*	Fortune's Drynaria Rhizome
gǔ qián	古錢			Old coins
guā dì	瓜蒂	*Pedicellus Melonis*		Melon stalk
tián guā dì	甜瓜蒂			
guàn zhòng	貫眾	*Rhizoma of Dryopteris Crassirhizomatis*	*Dryopteris crassirhizoma*	Wood fern
guī bǎn	龜板	*Carapax et Plastrum Testudinis*	*Chinemys reevesii*	Tortoise shell
guì yú	鱖魚		*Siniperca chuatsi* (Basilewsky)	Mandarin fish
guì yuán ròu	桂圓肉	*Arillus Longan*	*Dimocarpus longan* Lour.	Dried longan pulp
lóng yǎn ròu	龍眼肉			
guì zhī	桂枝	*Ramulus Cinnamomi*	*Cinnamomum cassia* Presl	Cassia twig
hǎi piāo xiāo	海螵蛸	*Endoconcha Sepiae*	*Sepiella maindroni de Rochebrune*	Cuttlebone

起
死
回
生

187

hān zǐ ké	蚶子殼	*Concha Arcae*	*Scapharca subcrenata; Arca subcrenata* Lischke.	Blood clam shells
wǎ léng zǐ	瓦楞子			
hé táo	核桃	*Semen Juglandis Regiae*	*Juglans regia*	English walnut
hú táo	胡桃			
hè shī	鶴虱	*Fructus Carpesii*	*Carpesium abrotanoides* (L.)	Common carpesium fruit
hēi dòu	黑豆	*Semen Glycine Macis*	*Glycine max* (L.)	Black bean
hēi dà dòu	黑大豆			
hóng fàn dòu	紅飯豆	*Semen Phaseoli*	*Vigna umbellata; Phaseolus calcaratus.*	Red rice beans (Adzuki bean)
chì xiǎo dòu	赤小豆			
hóng huā	紅花	*Flos Carthami*	*Carthamus tinctorius* (L.)	Safflower
hóng qū	紅麴	*Fermentum Rubrum*	*Monascus purpureus* Went.	Red food dye made from yeast.
hóng táng	紅糖			Brown sugar
hóng zǎo	紅棗	*Fructus Jujubae*	*Ziziphus jujuba*	Dried red Jujubes
hòu pò	厚朴	*Cortex Magnoliae Officinalis*	*Magnolia officinalis*	Officinal magnolia bark
hú jiāo	胡椒	*Fructus Piperis*	*Piper nigrum* (L.)	Pepper fruit
hú huáng lián	胡黃連	*Rhizoma Picrorhizae*	*Picrorhiza scrophularii flora* Pennell	Figwort flower picrorhiza rhizome
hǔ zhàng	虎杖	*Rhizoma et Radix Polygoni Cuspidati*	*Polygonum cuspidatum*	Giant knotweed rhizome
huā jiāo	花椒	*Pericarpium Zanthoxyli*	*Zanthoxylum bungeanum*	Prickly ash peel
huá shí	滑石		*Talcum*	Talc
huái huā	槐花	*Flos Sophorae*	*Sophora japonica* (L.)	Pagodatree flower
huái shān yào	淮山藥	*Rhizome Dioscoreae*	*Dioscorea opposita*	Common Yam Rhizome
huáng bǎi	黃柏	*Cortex Phellodendri*	*Phellodendron chinense*	Amur Corktree Bark
huáng dān	黃丹	*Plumbum Rubrum*		Red lead
huáng jīng yè	黃荊葉	*Folium Viticis Negundo*	*Vitex negundo* (L.)	Negundo Chastetree Leaf
huáng lián	黃連	*Rhizoma Coptidis*	*Coptis chinensis* Franch	
huáng qín	黃芩	*Radix Scutellariae*	*Scutellaria baicalensis* Georgi	baical skullcap root
huáng táng	黃糖			light brown sugar

188

huáng tǔ	黄土			a place with yellow earth [loess] is the best
huò xiāng	藿香	*Herba Agastaches*	*Agastache rugosa*	Wrinkled Giant hyssop
jiāng	薑	*Rhizoma Zingiberis*	*Zingiber officinale* Roscoe	Ginger
gān jiāng	乾薑			Dried ginger
lǎo jiāng	老薑			Old ginger
pào jiāng	炮薑			Blast-fried ginger
shēng jiāng	生薑			Fresh ginger
jiāng cán	僵蠶	*Bombyx Batryticatus*	*Bombyx mori* Linnaeus.	Silkworm
jiàng yóu	醬油			Soy sauce
jié gěng	桔梗	*Radix Platycodonis*	*Platycodon grandiforus*	Balloon flower
jiè cài zǐ	芥菜子	*Semen Brassicae Junceae*	*Brassica juncea*	Mustard seeds
jīn máo gǒu jí	金毛狗脊	*Rhizoma Cibotii*	*Cibotium barometz*	Rhizome of golden chicken fern, woolly fern
jīn yín huā	金銀花	*Flos Lonicerae*	*Lonicera japonica* Thunb.	Honey-suckle bud and flower
jīng jiè	荊芥	*Herba Schizonepetae*	*Schizonepeta tenuifolia*	Fine leaf schizonepeta herb
jiǔ cài	韭菜		*Allium tuberosum*	Chinese leeks
kǔ shēn	苦參	*Radix Sophorae Flavescentis*	*Sophora flavescens* Ait.	Light yellow sophora root
kuǎn dōng huā	款冬花	*Flos Farfarae*	*Tussilago farfara* (L.)	Common coltsfoot
lán diàn	藍靛	*Indigo Naturalis*	*Isatis tinctoria* (L.)	Indigo residue
qīng diàn	青靛			
léi wán	雷丸	*Omphalia*	*Polyporus mylittae; Mylitta lapidescens; Omphalia lapidescens*	Thunder ball
lí lú	藜蘆	*Radix et Rhizoma Veratri Nigri*	*Veratrum nigrum* (L.)	Black False Hellebore Root and Rhizome
lì zhī	荔枝	*Fructus Litchi*	*Litchi chinensis* Sonn.	Lychee
lì ròu	荔肉			Lychee flesh
lì zhī ròu	荔枝肉			Lychee flesh
lì zhī hé	荔枝核	*Semen Litchi*		Lychee pits
lián qiáo	連翹	*Fructus Forsythiae*	*Forsythia suspensa* (Thunb.) Vahl	Weeping forsythia capsule
liú huáng	硫黃		*Sulfur*	Sulfur

起
死
回
生

189

lóng yǎn hé	龍眼核	*Flos Longan*	*Dimocarpus longan* Lour.	Longan Flower
lú máo gēn	蘆茅根	*Rhizoma Phragmitis*	*Phragmites communis* Trin.	Rush rhizome
lú gēn	蘆根			
lǜ dòu	綠豆	*Semen Vignae Radiatae*	*Vigna radiata*	Mung bean
lù jiǎo	鹿角	*Cornu Cervi*	*Cervus nippon* Temminck	Deer horn; antler
luó bó	蘿蔔	*Radix Raphani*	*Raphanus sativus* (L.)	Radish
lái fú	萊菔			
mǎ chǐ xiàn	馬齒莧	*Herba Portulacae*	*Portulaca oleracea* (L.)	Purslane herb
mǎ dōu líng	馬兜鈴	*Fructus Aristolochiae*	*Aristolochia contorta*	Dutchman's-pipe fruit
mài dōng	麥冬	*Radix Ophiopogonis*	*Ophiopogon japonicus*	Dwarf lily turf tuber
mài fěn	麥粉			Wheat flour
méi tàn	煤炭			Coal
mù guā	木瓜	*Fructus Chaenomelis*	*Chaenomeles speciosa*	Flowering quince fruit
mù mián huā	木棉花	*Flos Bombacis*	*Bombax malabaricum*	Tree cotton flower
mù tàn pí	木炭皮			A thin 'skin' on the outside of a piece of charcoal
mù tōng	木通	*Caulis Akebiae*	*Akebia quinata*	Akebia stem
mù xiāng	木香	*Radix Aucklandiae*	*Aucklandia lappa* Decne.; *Saussurea lappa.*	Common aucklandia root
guǎng mù xiāng	廣木香			Common aucklandia root from Guǎngzhōu
nán guā ráng	南瓜瓤	*Pulpa Cucurbita moschata*	*Cucurbita moschata*	Pumpkin flesh
nán guā téng	南瓜藤	*Vitis Cucurbita moschata*	*Cucurbita moschata*	Pumpkin vine
nán péng shā	南硼砂		*Borax*	Borax
niú xī	牛膝	*Radix Achyranthis Bidentatae*	*Achyranthes bidentata* Bl.	Two toothed achyranthes root
ǒu	藕		*Nelumbo nucifera*	Lotus
hé huā	荷花	*Flos Nelumbinis*		Lotus flowers
hé yè	荷葉	*Folium Nelumbinis*		Lotus leaf
lián péng	蓮蓬	*Semen Nelumbinis*		Lotus seed pod
lián zǐ	蓮子	*Semen Nelumbinis*		Lotus seed pod

ǒu zhī	藕汁	Rhizoma Nelumbinis Nuciferae Recens		Fresh lotus root juice
pú gōng yīng	蒲公英	Herba Taraxaci	Taraxacum mongolicum	Dandelion leaf
qián hú	前胡	Radix Peucedani	Peucedanum praeruptorum Dunn.	Root of Whiteflower Hogfennel
qiàn shí	芡實	Semen Euryales	Euryale ferox Salisb.	Gordon euryale seed
qiāng huó	羌活	Rhizoma et Radix Notopterygii	Notopterygium incisum Ting.	Incised notopterygium rhizome and root
qiāng láng	蜣螂	Catharsius Molossus	Catharsius molossus	Dung beetle (scarab beetle)
qīng fěn	輕粉	Calomelas	Hg_2Cl_2	Calomel
qīng hāo	青蒿	Herba Artemisiae Annuae	Artemisia annua (L.)	Leaf of sweet wormwood
qīng yán	青鹽		Halitum	Halite
qīng xiāng zǐ huā	青葙子花	Semen Celosiae	Celosia argentea (L.)	Feather cockscomb seed
cǎo jué míng huā	草決明花			
qiū yǐn	蚯蚓	Pheretima	Pheretima aspergillum	Earthworms
qiū yǐn fèn	蚯蚓糞	Pheretima	Pheretima aspergillum	Earthworm excrement (castings)
ròu guì	肉桂	Cortex Cinnamomi	Cinnamomum cassia Presl.	Cinnamon bark
rǔ xiāng	乳香	Olibanum	Boswellia carterii Birdw.	Frankincense
sān léng	三棱	Rhizoma Sparganii	Spaganium stoloniferum	Common buried rubber
sān qī	三七	Radix Notoginseng	Panax notoginseng	
sāng shù zhī	桑樹枝	Ramulus Mori	Morus alba (L.)	Mulberry branches
sāng yè	桑葉	Folium Mori	Morus alba (L.)	Mulberry leaves
shā rén	砂仁	Fructus Amomi	Amomum villosum Lour.	Cardomum
yán shā rén	鹽砂仁			Salted cardomum
shā yuàn	沙苑	Semen Astragali Complanati	Astragalus complanatus	Astragalus seed
shān dòu gēn	山荳根	Radix Sophorae Tonkinensis	Sophora tonkinensis	Vietnamese sophora root
shān mù	杉木		Cunninghamia lanceolata	Chinese fir wood
shān mù tàn	杉木炭			Chinese fir wood charcoal

起
死
回
生

191

Pinyin	Chinese	Latin (Fructus/Radix)	Botanical	English
shān zhá	山查	Fructus Crataegi	Crataegus pinnatifida var. major N. E. Br.	Hawthorn fruit
jiāo [shān] zhá ròu	焦[山]查肉			Parched hawthorn fruit
shāo jiǔ	燒酒			White distilled liquor
shè xiāng	麝香	Moschus	Moschus berezovskii Flerov., M. sifanicus Przewalski	Musk
dāng mén zǐ	當門子			High quality shè xiāng.
shén qū	神麴	Massa Medicata Fermentata		Medicated leaven
shēng qí	生芪	Radix Astragali Recens	Astragalus membranaceus	
shēng huáng qí	生黃芪			
shēng míng fán	生明礬	Alumen Recens	Alunite	Fresh Alum
shēng shǒu wū	生首烏	Radix Polygoni Multiflori Recens	Polygonum multiflorum	Solomon's Seal
hé shǒu wū	何首烏			
shēng xuán fù huā gēn	生旋覆花根	Radix Inulae Recens	Inula japonica Thunb.	Fresh root of Japanese Inula, root of Linearleaf Inula, root of British Inula
shí dà gōng láo yè	十大功勞葉	Folium Mahoniae	Mahonia bealei	Leaf of Leatherleaf Mahonia, Leaf of Chinese Mahonia, Leaf of Japanese Mahonia
shǔ pà cǎo	鼠怕草			
shú shí gāo	熟石膏	Cooked Gypsum Fibrosum	Gypsum	Cooked gypsum
sī guā	絲瓜	Fructus Luffae	Luffa cylindrica	Luffa gourd
sōng huā	松花	Pollen Pini	Pinus massoniana	Pine pollen
sōng huā fēn	松花粉			
sōng xiāng	松香	Resin Pini	Pinus massoniana	Pine resin
sū hé xiāng	蘇合香	Styrax	Liquidambar orientalis Mill.	Storax, Storesin, Oriental Sweetgum
sū mù	蘇木	Lignum Sappan	Caesalpinia sappan (L.)	
sù ké	粟殼	Pericarpium Papaveris	Papaver somniferrum	Poppy husks
yīng sù ké	罌粟殼			
tán xiāng	檀香	Lignum Santali Albi	Santalum album (L.)	Sandal wood

táo rén	桃仁	*Semen Amygdali*	*Amygdalus persica* (L.)	Peach kernel
táo zhī jiān	桃枝尖	*Ramulus Amygdali*	*Amygdalus persica* (L.)	Peach twig tips
tiān dōng	天冬	*Radix Asparagi*	*Asparagus cochinchinensis*	
tiān má	天麻	*Rhizoma Gastrodiae*	*Gastrodia elata* Bl.	Tall gastrodia tuber
míng tiān má	明天麻			
tiān nán xīng	天南星	*Rhizoma Arisaematis*	*Arisaema erubescens*	Jack-in-the-pulpit tuber
shēng nán xīng	生南星			Fresh
tián jiǔ	甜酒			Sweet liquor
tián zhōng ní	田中泥			Mud from the center of a field
tiáo shēn	條參	*Radix Glehniae*	*Glehnia littoralis*	Coastal glehnia root
běi shā shēn	北沙參			
tiě zhā	鐵渣			Iron dust
tóng biàn	童便			Child's urine
tóng yóu	桐油	*Oleum Aleuritis Seminis*	*Aleurites fordii* Hemsl. (*Vernica fordii*)	Tung oil
tǔ biē chóng	土鱉蟲		*Eupolyphagia seu Steleophaga*	Ground beetle
tǔ fú líng	土茯苓	*Rhizoma Smilacis Glabrae*	*Smilax glabra* Roxb.	Glabrous greenbrier rhizome
tǔ gǒu	土狗		*Gryllotalpa*	mole cricket bugs, also called *lóu gǔ* 蝼蛄
tǔ gǒu chóng	土狗蟲			
wēi líng xiān	威靈仙	*Radix et Rhizoma Clematidis*	*Clematis chinensis*	Chinese clematis root
wū méi	烏梅	*Fructus Mume*	*Armeniaca mume*; *Prunus mume*	Smoked plum
wú gōng	蜈蚣	*Scolopendra*	*Scolopendra subspinipes mutilans*	Centipede
wú yí	蕪夷	*Fructus Ulmi Macrocarpae Preparatus*	*Ulmus macrocarpa*	Large-fruited Elm
wǔ líng zhī	五靈脂	*Faeces Trogopterori*	*Trogopterus xanthipes*	Flying squirrels droppings
xì xīn	細辛	*Herba Asari*	*Asarum heterotropoides; A. sieboldii.*	Manchurian wildginger

起
死
回
生

193

xiān táo cǎo	仙桃草	*Herba Veronicae Peregrinae*	*Veronica peregrina* (L.)	Neckweed, purslane speedwell
xiāng fù	香附	*Rhizoma Cyperi*	*Cyperus rotundus* (L.)	Nutgrass galingale rhizome
jiāng xiāng fù	薑香附			Ginger prepared
xiāng rú	香薷	*Herba Moslae*	*Mosla chinensis* Maxim.	Chinese mosla leaf
xīn chū jiào shí huī	新出窖石灰	*Lime*	*Lime*	Newly-emitted lime
xìng rén	杏仁	*Semen Armeniacae Amarum*	*Armeniaca vulgaris* Lam.	Bitter apricot kernel
kǔ xìng rén	苦杏仁			
xìng shù pí	杏樹皮	*Cortex Armeniacae Amarum*	*Armeniaca vulgaris* Lam.	Apricot tree bark
xióng huáng	雄黃		*Realgar*	Realgar
míng xióng	明雄			Lucid realgar
xuán fù huā	旋覆花	*Flos Inulae*	*Inula japonica* Thunb.	Inula flower
xuè jié	血竭	*Sanguis Darconis*	*Daemonorops draco*	Dragon's blood
yā piàn huī	鴉片灰			Opium ash
yàn xiāo	焰硝			Niter
xiāo shí	硝石			
yáng jìng gǔ	羊脛骨	*Os Caprae seu Ovis*	*Caprae seu Ovis*	Sheep [or goat] shin bone
yáng méi shù pí	楊梅樹皮		*Myrica rubra*	Chinese bayberry
yě jú huā	野菊花	*Flos Dendranthema indici*	*Dendranthema indicum* (L.) Des Moul.	Flower of Indian Dendranthema; Wild chrysanthemum
yì mǔ cǎo	益母草	*Herba Leonuri*	*Leonurus japonicus* Houtt.	Motherwort herb
yì yǐ rén	薏苡仁	*Semen Coicis*	*Coix lachryma-jobi* (L.)	Coix Seed
yǐ mǐ	苡米			
yīn chén	茵陳	*Herba Artemisiae Scopariae*	*Artemisia scoparia*	Virgate wormwood herb
yù tóu	芋頭	*Rhizoma Colocasiae Esculentae*	*Colocasia esculenta*	Taro
yù zān huā gēn	玉簪花根	*Radix Hosta Plantaginea*	*Hosta plantaginea*	Plantain lily root
yuán shēn	元參	*Radix Scrophulariae*	*Scrophularia ningpoensis*	Chinese figwort
xuán shēn	玄參			

194

yuè jì huā	月季花	Flos Rosae Chinensis	Rosa chinensis	Chinese rose
yuè yuè hóng	月月紅			
yún líng	雲苓	Poria	Poria cocos	Indian bread; Tuckahoe
zào jiá zǐ	皂荚子	Semen Gleditsiae	Gleditsia sinensis	Chinese Honeylocust seed
zào jiǎo	皂角	Spina Gleditsiae	Gleditsia sinensis	Chinese Honeylocust thorn
zé xiè	澤瀉	Rhizoma Alismatis	Alisma orientale	Oriental water plantain rhizome
zhāng mù	樟木	Lignum Cinnamomi Camphorae	Cinnamomum camphora	Camphor wood
zhāng shù yè	樟樹葉	Folium Cinnamomi Camphorae	Cinnamomum camphora	Camphor tree leaves
zhāng shù zǐ	樟樹子	Semen Cinnamomi Camphorae	Cinnamomum camphora	Camphor tree seeds
zhī mǔ	知母	Rhizoma Anemarrhenae	Anemarrhena asphodeloides	Common anemarrhena rhizome
zhī rén	栀仁	Fructus Gardeniae	Gardenia jasminoides Ellis	Cape Jasmine Fruit
shān zhī	山栀			
zhī zhū	蜘蛛	Aranea Ventricosa	Aranea ventricosa	Spider
zhǐ qiào	枳殼	Fructus Aurantii	Citrus aurantium (L.)	Orange fruit
zhì qí	炙芪	Radix Astragali	Astragalus membranaceus	Mix-fried astragalus
zhū lán gēn	珠蘭根	Radix Chloranthi spicati	Chloranthus spicatus	Pearl orchid root
zhū shā	朱砂	Cinnabaris	Cinnabar	Cinnabar
chén shā	辰砂			
zhù má yè	苧麻葉	Folium Boehmeriae Niveae	Boehmeria nivea	Household rush leaves
zǐ bèi fú píng	紫背浮萍	Herba Spirodelae	Spirodela polyrrhiza	Common Duckweed Herb
zǐ huā dì dīng	紫花地丁	Herba Violae	Viola philipica Cav.	Tokyo violet herb
zǐ sū	紫蘇	Folium Perillae	Perilla frutescens (L.) Britt.	Perilla leaf
zǐ sū yè	紫蘇葉			
zì rán tong	自然銅	Pyritum	Pyrite	Pyrite

起死回生

回生丹 *Huí Shēng Dān* (**Return to Life Elixir**)

live *tǔ biē chóng*	活土鼈蟲	5 *qián*
zì rán tóng	自然銅	3 *qián*
genuine *rǔ xiāng*	真乳香	2 *qián*
genuine aged *xuè jié*	真陳血竭	2 *qián*
genuine *zhū shā*	真珠砂	2 *qián*
bā dòu	巴豆	2 *qián*
shè xiāng (dāng mén zǐ)	真麝香	3 *fēn*

This treats patterns such as injuries from falling, crushing, beatings, knives, guns, cutting the throat, hangings, death due to fright, and drowning. Even if there are severe injuries all over the whole body and the victim has already been dead for several days, it is only necessary that the body remains somewhat soft.

蘇合丸 *Sū Hé Wán* (**Storax Pill**)

sū hé xiāng	蘇合香		10g
ān xí xiāng	安息香	mix these with the honey for making honey pills	20g
dīng xiāng	丁香		20g
mù xiāng	木香		20g
tán xiāng	檀香		20g
xiāng fù	香附	prepared with liquor and vinegar	20g
bái zhú	白朮	stir-fried in earth	20g
hē zǐ	訶子	remove the pit	20g
bì bá	蓽茇		20g
bā jiǎo huí xiāng	八角茴香	grind these eight into a fine powder [in gray]	10g
zhū shā	朱砂	water grind or crush into an extremely fine powder	10g
bīng piàn	冰片	finely ground	10g
rǔ xiāng	乳香	finely ground	10g

196

Then grind all the ingredients together again with the powdered *bīng piàn* 冰片 and *rǔ xiāng* 乳香, sift, and mix evenly. Mix each hundred grams of powder with forty to sixty grams of honey (pre-mixed with *sū hé xiāng* 蘇合香 and *ān xí xiāng* 安息香). Make it into honey pills and coat or wrap them up.

This pill dispels wind, settles pain, frees the orifices, and eliminates phlegm. It treats wind-phlegm reversal, stupor, loss of consciousness, pediatric convulsions, and wind phlegm abdominal pain with vomiting and diarrhea. Take three grams of honey pills orally, twice a day. This pill is contraindicated for pregnant women.

紅棗丸 *Hóng Zǎo Wán* (Red Date Pill)

| *hóng zǎo* | 紅棗 | 3 *jīn* |
| *shān mù* | 杉木 | ash |

When cooked, peel off the skin and remove the seeds. Grind the ash from the *shān mù* into a fine powder. Blend evenly with the *hóng zǎo* pulp and make it into pills the size of a marble. This treats red bayberry [syphilitic] infection and toxic sores all over the body, including those from taking *qīng fěn* and other types of minerals.

Hóng zǎo can resolve toxins from elixir minerals. *Shān mù* is special for expelling invasion of damp-heat.

二味拔毒散 *Èr Wèi Bá Dú Sàn* (Two Ingredient Powder to Pull Out Toxins)

| *xióng huáng* | 雄黃 | powdered |
| *kū fán* | 枯礬 | |

It treats all types of toxic *chóng* bites. Whether there is swelling, pain, or itching, it will immediately stop when this formula is applied. Its effects are miraculously quick. Mix equal portions of powdered *xióng huáng* and *kū fán*. First clean the site with ginger juice, mix the powder with tea and apply it.

紅膏藥 *Hóng Gāo Yào* (**Red Plaster**)

yín zhū	銀朱	water-grind, dry in the sun	1 *qián*
bì má rén	蓖麻仁		2 *qián*
nèn sōng xiāng	嫩松香		5 *qián*
huáng dān	黃丹	water-grind, dry in the sun	1 *qián*
qīng fěn	輕粉		5 *fēn*

Pound the above together until it is the consistency of mud and apply it. It draws out toxins, and treats clove sores, scrofula, and all types of toxic swellings. It also removes things that have become embedded in the flesh, such as metal, bamboo, wood, tile, and stone. When first applied, it may be a little painful and the patient may feel vexed and agitated, but the text says this does not indicate a problem.

托裏解毒湯 *Tuō Lǐ Jiě Dú Tāng* (**Expel Pus and Resolve Toxins Decoction**)

jīn yín huā	金銀花	2 *qián*
dāng guī	當歸	5 *qián*
shēng huáng qí	生黃耆	2 *qián*
tiān huā fěn	天花粉	1.5 *qián*
lián qiáo	連翹	1.5 *qián*
huáng qín	黃芩	1.5 *qián*
chì sháo	赤芍	1.5 *qián*
dà huáng	大黃	1 *qián*
mǔ lì	牡蠣	1 *qián*
shēng gān cǎo	生甘草	1 *qián*
zhǐ qiào	枳殼	6 *fēn*
zào cì	皂刺	0.5 *qián*

Boil the above in water and take it. This formula treats red swollen abscess-toxins. If the abscess has already broken open, remove the 皂刺 *zào cì*.

六一散 *Liù Yī Sàn* (Six-To-One Powder)

huá shí	滑石	6 parts
gān cǎo	甘草	1 part

This formula clears summer heat and disinhibits dampness. Take six to nine grams each time by swallowing it with a liquid, or wrap it in gauze and decoct it. Take it once or twice a day.

荊防敗毒散 *Jīng Fáng Bài Dú Sǎn* (Schizonepita and Saposhnikovia Toxin-Vanquishing Powder)

jīng jiè	荊芥	1 *qián*
fáng fēng	防風	1 *qián*
qiāng huó	羌活	1 *qián*
dú huó	獨活	1 *qián*
chái hú	柴胡	1 *qián*
qián hú	前胡	1 *qián*
chuān xiōng	川芎	1 *qián*
zhǐ qiào	枳殼	1 *qián*
jié gěng	桔梗	1 *qián*
fú líng	茯苓	1 *qián*
gān cǎo	甘草	5 *fēn*
bò hé	薄荷	3 *fēn*

Boil the above in water and take it. This treats swollen cheeks and fistulas of the cheeks.

十全大補湯 *Shí Quán Dà Bǔ Tāng* (Perfect Major Supplementation Decoction)

Grind together equal portions of:

rén shēn	人參
bái zhú	白朮

起死回生

fú líng	茯苓
zhì gān cǎo	炙甘草
shú dì huáng	熟地黃
bái sháo	白芍
dāng guī	當歸
chuān xiōng	川芎
ròu guì	肉桂
huáng qí	黃耆

Take two *qián* as a draft with three slices of ginger and two pieces of 大棗 *dà zǎo*. It warms and supplements qì and blood.

平胃散 *Píng Wèi Sàn* (Stomach-Calming Powder)
Finely powder together:

cāng zhú	蒼朮		5 *jīn*
hòu pǔ	厚樸	prepared with ginger juice and stir-fried until fragrant	3 *jīn* 2 *liǎng*
chén pí	陳皮		3 *jīn* 2 *liǎng*
gān cǎo	甘草	stir-fried	30 *liǎng*

Each dose is two *qián*. Place it in a small-cup of water with two slices of *shēng jiāng* (fresh ginger) and two pieces of *dà zǎo*. Boil it together down to seventy percent. Remove the ginger and *dà zǎo*, and take it while hot on an empty stomach. It treats disharmony of the spleen and stomach with loss of appetite, regulates qì, warms the stomach, transforms food accumulations, and disperses phlegm-rheum.

黃連解毒湯 *Huáng Lián Jiě Dú Tāng* (Coptis Toxin-Resolving Decoction)

huáng lián	黃連	3 *qián*
huáng qín	黃芩	2 *qián*

| huáng bǎi | 黃柏 | | 2 qián |
| zhī zǐ | 梔子 | split | 14 pcs |

Boil in six *shēng* of water down to two *shēng* and take it in two doses. It drains fire and resolves toxins.

解毒丸 *Jiě Dú Wán* (Resolve Toxins Pills)

bǎn lán gēn	板藍根	washed clean and sun-dried	120g
guàn zhòng	貫眾		30g
qīng dài	青黛	ground	30g
shēng gān cǎo	生甘草	split	14 pcs

Powder the above and make honey pills the size of *wú tóng* seeds. Coat them with *qīng dài*. Quickly take three to five pills, which should be about fifteen grams. Chew them and swallow with water. It clears heat and resolves toxins, and treats accidental overdose of toxic herbs or other toxic things, with stupor and nausea.

Pinyin Index

Medicinal Index

起
死
回
生

203

起死回生

起死回生

Formula Index

General Index

起死回生

起
死
回
生

起
死
回
生

213

起
死
回
生

215

The Chinese Medicine Database

www.cm-db.com

The Chinese Medicine Database has been organized around one central principle -- translation of Classical Chinese texts, and dissemination of that information.

There are thousands of Chinese medicine texts that have never been translated. We have compiled a small list on our website of the ones that we have found, but we believe that there are tens of thousands of documents that span from the *Hàn* Dynasty to pre-Republican times. Most of these documents will never be read by people in the West, simply because of lack of translation.

We have created a vehicle, that allows interested practitioners, students, institutions, and scholars to help support and fund the translation of these documents, and then mine and synthesize the data that is gained from these texts.

The Database contains:

Monographs on:
> 687 Single Herbs
> 1510 Formulas
> Mayway's Patents
> ITM's Formulations
> Golden Flowers Formulations
> Health Concerns Formulations
> Blue Poppy's Patents
> Classical Pearls Formulations by Heiner Fruehauf
> OBGYN Modifications to Formulas
> Single Points: the 361 Regular Points

Beer Hall Lecture Series
> Watch videos from our monthly Beer Hall lecture series with guest speakers such as: Arnaud Versluys, Subhuti Dharmananda, Jason Robertson, Craig Mitchell, Michael Max, Lorraine Wilcox, and Ed Neal.

Play STORT
> Play our free online game STORT where you can learn Chinese while having a bit of fun (www.cm-db.com/stort).

15,000 Western Diagnoses with ICD-9 Codes

起
死
回
生

A Chinese-English dictionary:
Containing over 101,368 terms, including the Eastland and the WHO term sets.

A Western Book search containing:
Fenner's Complete Formulary
    by B. Fenner
The 1918 Dispensatory of the United States of America
    Edited by Joseph P. Remington, Horatio C. Woods and others
The Eclectic Materia Medica, Pharmacology and Therapeutics
    by Harvey Wickes Felter, M.D.

A Personal Dashboard, which allows users to:
Blog
Take notes on any monograph.
Search for other users by city, state, country and name.
Make friends all around the world.
Share and compare notes with friends.
Personalize your dashboard by adding photos, and information about your practice.

Translations:

Shāng Hán Lái Sū Jí	傷寒來蘇集	Renewal of Treatise on Cold Damage
Qí Jing Bā Mài Kǎo	奇經八脈考	Explanation of the Eight Vessels of the Marvellous Meridians
Shāng Hán Míng Lǐ Lùn	傷寒明理論	Treatise on Enlightening the Principles of Cold Damage
Wú Jū Tōng Yì Àn	吴鞠通医案	Case Studies of Wú Jūtōng
The Nàn Jīng	難經	The Classic of Difficulties
The Zàng Fǔ Biāo Běn Hán Rè Xū Shí Yòng Yào Shì	臟腑標本寒熱虛實用藥式	Viscera and Bowels, Tip and Root, Cold and Heat, Vacuity and Repletion Model for Using Medicinals
Wēn Rè Lún	温熱論	Treatise on Warm Heat Disease
Shāng Hán Shé Jiàn	傷寒舌鑒	Tongue Mirror of Cold Damage
Xǔ Shì Yì Àn	許氏醫案	Case Histories of Master Xǔ
Fǔ Xing Jué Zāng Fǔ Yòng Yào Fǎ Yào	輔行決臟腑用藥法要	Secret Instructions for Assisting the Body: Essential Methods for the Application of Drugs to the Viscera & Bowels
Biāo Yōu Fù	標幽賦	Indicating the Obscure

Liú Juān Zǐ Guǐ Yí Fāng	劉涓子鬼遺方	Liu Juanzi's Formulas Inherited from Ghosts
Shèn Jí Chú Yán	慎疾芻言	Precautions in Illness: My Humble Thoughts
Yào Zhèng Jì Yí	藥症忌宜	Medicinals & Patterns Contraindications & Appropriate [Choices]
Fù Kē Wèn Dá	婦科問答	Questions and Answers in Gynecology
Nèi Jīng Zhī Yào	內經知要	Essential Knowledge from the Nèijīng

Benefits:

Subscribers to the Database receive a 10% discount on our published books when they are in pre-release.

We translate texts as often, and in quantities that reflect our user base. The larger amount of subscribers that we have, the more translation that we can accomplish.

Published Books:

2008 Bèi Jí Qiān Jīn Yào Fāng 備急千金要方: Essential Prescriptions Worth a Thousand Gold Pieces For
   Emergencies. vol. 2-4 by Sūn Sīmiǎo 孫思邈
   Translated by Sabine Wilms.
   ISBN 978-0-9799552-0-4

2010 Zhēn Jiǔ Dà Chéng 針灸大成: The Great Compendium of Acupuncture & Moxabustion vol. I by
   Yáng Jìzhōu 楊繼洲
   Translated by Sabine Wilms.
   ISBN 978-0-9799552-2-8

2010 Zhēn Jiǔ Dà Chéng 針灸大成: The Great Compendium of Acupuncture & Moxabustion vol. V by
   Yáng Jìzhōu 楊繼洲
   Translated by Lorraine Wilcox.
   ISBN 978-0-9799552-4-2

2010 Jīn Guì Fāng Gē Kuò 金匱方歌括: Formulas from the Golden Cabinet with Songs vol. I - III by
  Chén Xiūyuán 陳修園
  Translated by Sabine Wilms.
  ISBN 978-0-9799552-5-9

2011 Zhēn Jiǔ Dà Chéng 針灸大成: The Great Compendium of Acupuncture & Moxabustion vol. VIII by
  Yáng Jìzhōu 楊繼洲
  Translated by Yue Lu.
  ISBN 978-0-9799552-7-3

2011 Zhēn Jiǔ Dà Chéng 針灸大成: The Great Compendium of Acupuncture & Moxabustion vol. IX by
  Yáng Jìzhōu 楊繼洲
  Translated by Lorraine Wilcox.
  ISBN 978-0-9799552-6-6

起
死
回
生

CPSIA information can be obtained
at www.ICGtesting.com
Printed in the USA
BVOW06s1120211117
500165BV00006BA/93/P